Gynaecology for the Obstetrician

Gynaecology for the Obstetrician

Edited by
Swati Jha
Sheffield Teaching Hospitals NHS FT

Priya Madhuvrata
Sheffield Teaching Hospitals NHS FT

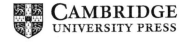

CAMBRIDGE
UNIVERSITY PRESS

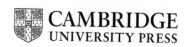

Shaftesbury Road, Cambridge CB2 8EA, United Kingdom

One Liberty Plaza, 20th Floor, New York, NY 10006, USA

477 Williamstown Road, Port Melbourne, VIC 3207, Australia

314–321, 3rd Floor, Plot 3, Splendor Forum, Jasola District Centre, New Delhi – 110025, India

103 Penang Road, #05–06/07, Visioncrest Commercial, Singapore 238467

Cambridge University Press is part of Cambridge University Press & Assessment, a department of the University of Cambridge.

We share the University's mission to contribute to society through the pursuit of education, learning and research at the highest international levels of excellence.

www.cambridge.org
Information on this title: www.cambridge.org/9781009208826

DOI: 10.1017/9781009208802

First published 2023

Printed in the United Kingdom by CPI Group Ltd, Croydon CR0 4YY

A catalogue record for this publication is available from the British Library.

Library of Congress Cataloging-in-Publication Data
Names: Jha, Swati, editor. | Madhuvrata, Priya, editor.
Title: Gynaecology for the obstetrician / edited by Swati Jha, Sheffield
   Teaching Hospitals NHS FT, Priya Madhuvrata, Sheffield Teaching
   Hospitals NHS FT.
Description: Cambridge, United Kingdom ; New York, NY : Cambridge
   University Press, 2023. | Includes bibliographical references and index.
Identifiers: LCCN 2023001229 (print) | LCCN 2023001230 (ebook) |
   ISBN 9781009208826 (paperback) | ISBN 9781009208802 (epub)
Subjects: LCSH: Pregnancy–Complications. | Generative organs,
   Female–Diseases. | Gynecology.
Classification: LCC RG571 .G96 2023 (print) | LCC RG571 (ebook) |
   DDC 618.2–dc23/eng/20230309
LC record available at https://lccn.loc.gov/2023001229
LC ebook record available at https://lccn.loc.gov/2023001230

ISBN 978-1-009-20882-6 Paperback

This book is dedicated to all my past teachers and trainers who instilled in me my passion for the specialty and all past and current trainees who make me want to continue teaching
Swati Jha
Sheffield

Dedicated to all mothers who have sustained ante-natal, intrapartum and post-natal gynaecological morbidity and to my lovely husband Madhu and children, Anshu and Adi
Priya Madhuvrata
Sheffield

Contents

Contributors

Parveen Abedin (FRCOG), Consultant Gynaecologist and Unit Lead for Gynaecological Oncology, Birmingham Women's & Children's Hospital, UK

Juliet Albert (BA (Hons), BSc (Hons), RGN, RM, MSc, FRCM), FGM Specialist Midwife and FGM Trust Lead, The Sunflower Clinics, Imperial College Healthcare NHS Trust, London, UK

Lina Antoun (MD, MRCOG), Specialist Registrar and Clinical Research Fellow, Birmingham Women's NHS Foundation Trust/University of Birmingham, UK

Claire Baldry, Consultant Clinical Oncologist, Weston Park Hospital, Sheffield, UK

Helen Bolton (DLM, PhD, MRCOG), Consultant in Gynaecology and Gynaecological Oncology, Cambridge University Hospitals NHS Foundation Trust, Addenbrooke's Hospital, Cambridge, UK

T. Justin Clark (MD, FRCOG), Consultant Gynaecologist and Honorary Professor, Birmingham Women's NHS Foundation Trust/University of Birmingham, UK

Mary Connor (MD, FRCOG, MSc Advanced Gynaecological Endoscopy), Consultant Gynaecologist, Department of Obstetrics and Gynaecology, Sheffield Teaching Hospitals NHS Foundation Trust, UK; Honorary Senior Lecturer, Obstetrics and Gynaecology, University of Sheffield, UK

Emma Ferriman, Consultant Obstetrician and Gynaecologist, Sheffield Teaching Hospitals NHS Foundation Trust, UK

Charlotte Gatenby (MBChB), Specialty Trainee Year 4, CSRH Norwich, iCaSH, UK

Neil Harvey (MBChB, FRCS(Urol)), Consultant Urological Surgeon, Royal Bolton Hospital, Bolton NHS Foundation Trust, Greater Manchester, UK

Swati Jha (MD, FRCOG), Consultant Gynaecologist and Honorary Professor, Sheffield Teaching Hospitals NHS Foundation Trust/University of Sheffield, UK

Rohna Kearney (MD, FRCOG), Consultant Urogynaecologist, Saint Mary's Hospital, Manchester University NHS Foundation Trust, UK; Honorary Senior Lecturer, University of Manchester, UK

Pallavi Latthe (MD, FRCOG, DFFP, Cert Med Ed), O&G Consultant, Subspecialist in Urogynaecology, Clinical Lead for Paediatric and Adolescent Gynaecology, Birmingham Women's and Children's NHS Foundation Trust, UK

Priya Madhuvrata (MBBS, MD, FRCOG), Consultant Obstetrician and Gynaecologist, Sheffield Teaching Hospitals NHS Foundation Trust, UK; Honorary Senior Lecturer, Obstetrics and Gynaecology, University of Sheffield, UK

Jenna Morgan, Oncoplastic Breast Surgeon, Doncaster and Bassetlaw Teaching Hospitals NHS Foundation Trust, South Yorkshire, UK

David Nunns (MD FRCOG), Consultant Gynaecological Oncologist, Nottingham University Hospitals NHS Trust, UK

Nicola Adanna Okeahialam (MBChB, MD), Urogynaecology Clinical Research Fellow, Croydon University Hospital, Thornton Heath, UK

Julia E. Palmer (MD, FRCOG), Consultant Gynaecological Oncologist, Sheffield Teaching Hospitals NHS Foundation Trust, UK

Victoria L. Parker (PhD, MCROG), Speciality Registrar in Obstetrics and Gynaecology, Sheffield Teaching Hospitals NHS Foundation Trust, UK; NIHR Clinical Lecturer in Obstetrics and Gynaecology, The University of Sheffield, UK

Ian Pearce (B Med Sci, BMBS, FCRS (Urol)), Consultant Urological Surgeon, Manchester Royal Infirmary, Manchester University NHS Foundation Trust, UK; Honorary Professor, Salford University, UK; Honorary Senior Lecturer, University of Manchester, UK

Bibi Zeyah Fatemah Sairally (MB ChB, MRCOG, FHEA, PgCert Med Ed), O&G Specialist Registrar, Warwick Hospital, UK

Catherine Schünmann (FRCOG, MFSRH), Consultant, SRH Norwich, iCaSH, UK

Abdul H. Sultan (MD, FRCOG), Consultant Obstetrician and Urogynaecologist, Croydon University Hospital, Thornton Heath, UK; Honorary Reader, St George's University of London, UK

Ranee Thakar (MD, FRCOG), Consultant Obstetrician and Urogynaecologist, Croydon University Hospital, Thornton Heath, UK; Honorary Senior Lecturer, St George's University of London, UK

Nikolaos Thanatsis (MD, PhD), Urogynaecology and Pelvic Floor Unit, University College London Hospital, UK

Arvind Vashisht (MA, MD, FRCOG), Urogynaecology and Pelvic Floor Unit, University College London Hospital, UK

Lynda Wyld, Professor of Surgical Oncology, University of Sheffield, UK; Consultant Oncoplastic Breast Surgeon, Doncaster and Bassetlaw Teaching Hospitals NHS Foundation Trust, South Yorkshire, UK

Masha Ben Zvi (MD), Urogynaecology and Pelvic Floor Unit, University College London Hospital, UK

Foreword

In this era of medical specialisation, we are increasingly becoming skilled at our jobs and deskilled in managing areas out with our specialist expertise. The Royal College of Obstetricians and Gynaecologist's *High Quality Women's Health Care* report of 2011 proposed a number of changes needed in the education and training of doctors in the specialty of obstetrics and gynaecology. As a result, the *Advanced Training in Obstetrics and Gynaecology* document was published in August 2019, which addresses the purpose, learning outcomes and content of learning, in addition to the core curriculum requirement for the Certificate of Completion of Training (CCT). Neither the core curriculum nor the obstetric Advanced Training Skills Modules (ATSMs – Advanced labour ward; Fetal medicine; High-risk pregnancy; Labour ward lead; Obstetric medicine) include management of the complex gynaecological problems encountered commonly during pregnancy or in the post-natal period. And yet, obstetricians who have completed the above-listed obstetric ATSMs would be expected to competently manage women with complex gynaecological problems. This book provides the knowledge base to improve the quality of care provided to pregnant and post-natal women suffering from complex gynaecological problems. It will help to manage patient expectations and thereby improve patient satisfaction. It will also help decrease complaints, litigation and claims by providing appropriate management and protocols. And last but not least, it will be hugely beneficial to obstetricians working within and outside the UK who are managing common and less common gynaecological problems that occur in pregnancy.

I welcome this unique new book which is the first to address this important area so comprehensively. I believe it will play a significant role in equipping colleagues with the skills needed to manage pregnant women and will drive improvements in both patient safety and the prevention of adverse events.

I commend the efforts of all the contributors to this book, which provides us with an evidence-based approach to the management of gynaecological problems in our obstetric practice. It is a valuable addition to the women's health literature.

Dame Lesley Regan
Professor of Obstetrics and Gynaecology, Imperial College London;
Honorary Consultant, St Mary's Hospital, London;
Past President, RCOG

Preface

There was a time when the terms obstetrician or gynaecologist were used interchangeably; however, in this day and age of specialisation, we are becoming increasingly skilled at managing medical problems within our remit of practice, and deskilled at those out with. The role of a consultant has evolved with the increasing challenges of scientific progress and rapid development in clinical practice, service delivery and working patterns. Increased years of training within a specialty has its obvious advantages and makes us better at what we do. Specialisation has meant that in making professional decisions pertaining to our branch of medicine, the buck stops with us. This is believed to give better job satisfaction and assure quality, as we are working in an area we are passionate about. It also instils greater trust from our patients. Malcolm Gladwell rightly observed in his book, *Outliers: The Story of Success*, that the key is the ten-thousand-hour rule. Excellence at performing complex tasks requires a critical minimum level of practice over and over again, and research has shown that this is the magic number of hours required to be an expert. By extrapolation, however, this also implies that being an expert in multiple areas is hugely unlikely.

Looking beyond obstetrics and gynaecology, we see this in other specialities too. For example, within orthopaedics, specialisation is linked to different joints. So, we have the ankle, shoulder, knee, hip and spine orthopods. Increasingly we are becoming technicians who service a specific organ.

This is in part because medical knowledge is ever expanding, and it would be impossible to keep up. However, most clinicians have this insight and are therefore more willing to have robust discussions about the diagnosis, options for management and care of their patients who have other underlying conditions, which they themselves are not experts at managing. This curiosity and interest beyond one's own area of expertise shows both maturity and wisdom.

Some preliminary research has shown that splitting the specialities of obstetrics and gynaecology may make both specialities more attractive, with better recruitment and retention. However, at least for the foreseeable future, the two specialities are inextricably linked. The beauty of our specialty is that it combines both medicine and surgery, which has a strong appeal to those joining, and to this day, a majority of those practising within the specialty practise both. However, even then, for those inclined more towards one area, there can arise clinical scenarios that we are uncomfortable managing as these are not seen on a regular day-to-day basis.

The purpose of the book is to cover all aspects of gynaecological problems encountered by obstetricians during the antenatal, intrapartum and post-natal periods. Although a balance between increasing specialisations and workforce limits can be achieved through local and regional networks, this book will be invaluable in managing complex clinical scenarios and clinical dilemmas encountered in our day-to-day practice with high-quality evidence resulting in safe and effective care with good governance. This will benefit obstetricians across the globe as neither the standard obstetrics and gynaecology textbooks nor the curriculum cover the topics included in our book in such a detailed manner. In each chapter we have provided details of issues of governance that need to be taken into account. This will enable obstetricians to provide evidence-based counselling as well as manage and make appropriate referrals to improve the quality of care provided and clinical outcomes, while simultaneously reducing patient dissatisfaction, complaints and litigation.

Professor Swati Jha
Dr Priya Madhuvrata
Sheffield Teaching Hospitals NHS Foundation Trust

Chapter 1

Ovarian Cysts in Pregnancy

Masha Ben Zvi, Nikolaos Thanatsis, Arvind Vashisht

1.1 Introduction

Although the assessment and management of ovarian cysts in non-pregnant women has been studied extensively, unfortunately the same does not apply to the pregnant population. It is difficult to be certain about the exact incidence of ovarian cysts complicating pregnancy, and rates reportedly vary between 0.05–6% [1]. Their prevalence decreases with advanced gestational age, likely due to spontaneous resolution of physiological ovarian cysts.

Historically, ovarian cysts were diagnosed prenatally if they were large enough to be palpated, or they might be an incidental finding during a Caesarean section. The widespread use of ultrasound in early pregnancy and antenatal surveillance has led to an increase in the diagnosis of ovarian cysts during pregnancy. Fortunately, most of them are benign and will resolve spontaneously during the antenatal period. Nevertheless, even benign cysts can generate symptoms and become a source of anxiety, both for patients and for their physicians. In addition, a small proportion of ovarian cysts in pregnancy (about 1–5%) will carry some malignant potential [2, 3]. Hence, early identification, appropriate diagnostic work-up and optimal management are necessary, of course taking into consideration the complexities arising from the pregnant status of the patients.

This chapter serves to summarise current evidence for the assessment and management of ovarian cysts in pregnancy. Key concepts such as counselling, optimal time to operate and post-natal follow-up are also discussed.

1.2 Types of Cysts

Similarly to non-pregnant women, ovarian cysts identified in pregnancy can be broadly divided into three categories: benign, malignant and borderline cysts. About 95–99% of them are benign, while malignant (most commonly germ cell, sex cord stromal and epithelial tumours) and borderline cysts (predominantly serous and mucinous borderline tumours) account for approximately 1–5% and 1–2% of the ovarian cysts diagnosed in pregnancy, respectively [2, 3].

Most ovarian cysts are functional in nature with the corpus luteum being the most commonly encountered cyst in pregnancy [4]; functional ovarian cysts may also represent simple follicular or haemorrhagic cysts. The most usual benign, non-functional cysts are endometriomas, mature teratomas (dermoid cysts) and serous or mucinous cystadenomas or cystadenofibromas. The above cysts demonstrate distinct ultrasound features and are usually readily identifiable by an experienced sonologist.

Table 1.1 The most common types of ovarian cysts and non-ovarian adnexal masses in pregnancy

Benign ovarian cysts	Corpus luteum and other functional cysts Endometrioma Dermoid cyst (mature teratoma) Serous cystadenoma Mucinous cystadenoma Cystadenofibroma
Primary malignant ovarian cysts	Germ cell tumour Epithelial ovarian cancer including borderline tumours Sex cord stromal tumours
Metastatic malignant ovarian tumours	Chiefly metastatic breast and gastrointestinal cancer
Benign non-ovarian adnexal masses	Hydrosalpinx-pyosalpinx Tubo-ovarian abscess Fimbrial or paratubal cyst Para-ovarian cyst Peritoneal inclusion cyst (pseudocyst) Pedunculated or broad ligament fibroid Appendiceal abscess or mucocele Diverticular abscess Pelvic kidney
Unique in pregnancy	Ectopic pregnancy

Table 1.1 summarises the most common types of ovarian cysts in pregnancy as well as some non-ovarian adnexal masses, which are essential to consider during differential diagnosis.

1.3 Clinical Presentation and Complications

Most pregnant women with ovarian cysts are asymptomatic; the cyst is actually an incidental finding either during a routine early pregnancy or antenatal ultrasound examination or during a Caesarean section. Usually, patients become symptomatic either when a cyst enlarges significantly and can be palpated through the abdomen or, more often, if a cyst complication occurs. Physicians should bear in mind that many cyst accident symptoms are non-specific and can easily be mistaken for common pregnancy symptoms (abdominal cramping and discomfort, nausea, vomiting); thus, leading to a delayed diagnosis and management of an acute complication [5]. Torsion, cyst rupture and haemorrhage are the usual cyst accidents both in non-pregnant and pregnant women. In addition, obstruction of labour by a very large ovarian cyst is a unique to pregnancy, albeit very rare, complication [6].

1.3.1 Torsion

Data on the incidence of ovarian torsion in pregnancy are conflicting, and rates in the literature vary from 0.1 to 15% [3, 4]. While an ovarian torsion may occur even in the absence of a cyst in women with elongated ovarian ligaments, the condition is more common if the ovary is enlarged and 'heavy', such as in the presence of large ovarian cysts especially those with solid components (e.g. dermoid cysts) or in ovarian hyperstimulation syndrome. Condous et al. estimated the overall risk of torsion at 0.1%, rising to 5–15% if an ovarian cyst coexists [4]. Approximately 10–20% among all cases of ovarian torsion take place during pregnancy, and 60% of them occur between 10–17 weeks gestation, likely due to cephalad displacement of the ovaries [7, 8]. Large ovarian cysts are also likely to undergo torsion during the early post-partum period; as the uterus involutes, more intra-abdominal space is available for a displaced ovary to undergo torsion.

The symptoms a pregnant woman with ovarian torsion will present with are similar to those of a non-pregnant woman: sudden-onset sharp abdominal pain, constant or intermittent in nature, radiating to the back, groin or flank, nausea, vomiting and occasionally anorexia. On examination, patients may display signs of peritonism, adnexal tenderness and cervical excitation [5].

Serum markers such as leucocytosis have a limited role in the diagnostic evaluation of pregnant women with a suspected ovarian torsion. On the contrary, transvaginal ultrasonography, with a reported positive predictive value of 87.5% and specificity of 93.3%, is the most useful diagnostic tool [9]. The most common sonographic features observed in ovarian torsion include enlargement of the ovary when compared to the contralateral one, oedema of the ovarian parenchyma and peripherally displaced follicles, perhaps along with transudation of fluid into the displaced follicles. The presence of a displaced ovary (e.g. at the uterine-vesico fold or even at the contralateral side of the pelvis) as well as the 'whirlpool sign' on colour Doppler examination (i.e. twisted vascular pedicle) are also useful ultrasound features raising the suspicion of ovarian torsion. Finally, free fluid in the pouch of Douglas can also be noticed in patients with ovarian torsion (as well as in women with ovarian cyst rupture; in the former event, the fluid is reactive in origin and usually its volume is significantly reduced compared to cases of a ruptured cyst).

If ultrasound examination is inconclusive, then MRI can be utilised to investigate a possible ovarian torsion in pregnant women. The use of gadolinium contrast medium should be avoided. On the contrary, CT has no place in the diagnostic work-up of pregnant patients with a suspected ovarian torsion [10].

It should be flagged that ovarian torsion remains a clinical diagnosis; even though ultrasound imaging is routinely used to aid diagnosis, clinical examination is still the diagnostic cornerstone, and a strong consideration is made to proceed to surgical intervention should the clinical findings be highly suspicious of ovarian torsion.

1.3.2 Ovarian Cyst Rupture and Haemorrhage

Rupture of an ovarian cyst and subsequent haemorrhage, or haemorrhage within an intact ovarian cyst, are quite common cyst accidents that may occur both in pregnant and non-pregnant women. Patients usually present with non-specific symptoms such as sudden-onset lower pelvic pain, nausea and vomiting; of note, pain tends to be worse at the onset of symptoms and may subside by the time of presentation. In the vast majority of cases, the associated haemorrhage is not clinically significant; patients are usually haemodynamically stable; symptoms are manageable with analgesia and tend to resolve within a few days. In the unlikely event of significant intra-abdominal bleeding though, women may present with hypovolemic shock and necessitate an acute surgical intervention.

Similar to ovarian torsion, ultrasound is the first-line imaging modality in suspected ovarian cyst rupture. An experienced sonologist can usually easily identify the presence of haemoperitoneum in the pelvis or even in the upper abdomen and hence, can assess the severity of intra-abdominal bleeding. Furthermore, haemorrhage within an intact ovarian cyst has distinct ultrasound features: a fresh blood clot may display a lace-like or spider-web appearance; it is avascular on Doppler examination and can be seen to 'wobble' in a jelly-like fashion on palpation with a transvaginal probe [5]. The ultrasound appearance of blood may be anechoic in early stages, whereas in later stages accumulated old blood may have a 'ground-glass' appearance as in an endometrioma.

1.3.3 Mass Effect: Obstruction of Labour

Like any large pelvic mass, should an ovarian cyst enlarge significantly, it may apply pressure to surrounding structures, including the urinary bladder, ureters, urethra and intestines. The associated symptoms vary and will be determined by which organ is affected and to what degree. The same mechanism is responsible for the obstruction of labour: if a large ovarian cyst is located adjacent to the lower uterine segment and below the presenting part, it may contribute to labour dystocia [10].

1.4 Diagnostic Evaluation

A thorough medical history and physical examination constitute the mainstay of assessment of pregnant women with ovarian cysts. Further tests such as a full blood count; renal, liver function and electrolytes; C-reactive protein (CRP); coagulation screen; as well as a urine dipstick/culture and triple vaginal swabs may also be useful depending on the clinical scenario, chiefly in acutely unwell patients presenting with suspected cyst accidents [5]. The diagnostic work-up would be incomplete without the use of imaging modalities to characterise the nature of the cyst, to discriminate between benign and malignant lesions, to investigate any possible acute cyst complications and to guide further management.

1.4.1 Imaging

Ultrasonography is considered the first-line imaging modality in pregnant women with an ovarian cyst [11]. It is safe both for the mother and the fetus, widely available and cheaper compared to alternative options; hence, it is an ideal primary evaluation tool.

Transvaginal ultrasound can be used as early as the fourth to fifth week of gestation to confirm the implantation site and exclude an extrauterine or heterotopic pregnancy. Assessment of the ovaries and the Fallopian tubes is becoming standard practice during an early pregnancy scan, allowing early identification of adnexal cysts, even if they are quite small and asymptomatic.

Accurate characterisation of the nature of ovarian cysts identified in pregnancy is crucial. Subjective pattern recognition (i.e. subjective impression of the sonologist) has a very good diagnostic performance for the assessment of adnexal cysts with a sensitivity and specificity equal to those of complex logistic regression models [12, 13]. However, this requires an expert ultrasound operator, and it remains questionable whether it can be safely applied to a non-expert setting [14]. As a result, many algorithms and models have been developed in an attempt to improve the diagnostic accuracy of non-expert

Table 1.2 The IOTA 'simple rules' and 'simple descriptors' for differentiation between malignant and benign adnexal lesions

Simple descriptors

Benign descriptors
- Unilocular tumour with ground-glass echogenicity in premenopausal women (suggestive of an endometrioma)
- Unilocular tumour with mixed echogenicity and acoustic shadows in premenopausal women (suggestive of a dermoid cyst)
- Unilocular cyst of anechoic content with regular walls and largest diameter less than 10 cm (suggestive of a simple cyst or a cystadenoma)
- Remaining unilocular tumours with regular walls (suggestive of functional cysts)

Malignant descriptors
- Tumour with ascites and at least moderate colour Doppler blood flow in postmenopausal women
- Women aged > 50 years and CA-125 > 100 IU/mL

Simple rules

Benign features	Malignant features
- Unilocular cyst	- Irregular solid tumour
- Largest diameter of largest solid component <7 mm	- Ascites
	- At least four papillary projections
- Acoustic shadows	- Irregular multilocular solid tumour with largest diameter ≥100 mm
- Smooth multilocular tumour with largest diameter <100 mm	- Very strong intratumoral blood flow on colour or power Doppler
- No intratumoral blood flow on colour or power Doppler	

examiners. Some of these models, such as the Risk of Malignancy Index (RMI), take into account other factors besides the ultrasound characteristics (e.g. cancer antigen-125 (CA-125)), some of which alter during pregnancy and hence, cannot be applied to pregnant women [13].

The International Ovarian Tumor Analysis (IOTA) group has published extensively on ultrasound-based models to differentiate between malignant and benign ovarian cysts. The group has proposed 'simple descriptors' and 'simple rules'. These help non-expert operators classify most ovarian lesions as benign or malignant with a reported sensitivity of 95% and specificity of 91%, leaving only a small proportion of indeterminate cases to be assessed by expert sonologists [15, 16]. Table 1.2 presents the IOTA 'simple rules' and 'simple descriptors' for differentiation between malignant and benign adnexal lesions [15].

The pregnant status of patients should always be kept in mind during an ultrasound evaluation of an ovarian cyst. Even benign cysts such as endometriomas may undergo major morphological changes during pregnancy, referred to as decidualisation, and mimic malignancy. The effect of pregnancy-related high progesterone levels on the ectopic endometrial tissue of an endometrioma results in the formation of ectopic decidua. Sonographically, a decidualised endometrioma is characterised by a thick, irregular inner wall and prominent intraluminal papillary projections with increased blood flow on Doppler examination, similar to malignant ovarian tumours. As shown by Pateman et al. [17], about 12% of endometriomas will undergo decidualisation during pregnancy. In such cases, ultrasound examiners should look for other features to confirm their benign nature, such as the presence of extraovarian nodules of deep infiltrating endometriosis (e.g. in the uterosacral ligaments, the rectovaginal space or the rectosigmoid colon), obliteration of the pouch of Douglas as well as the tendency of endometriomas to decrease in size and regress rapidly during pregnancy, contrary to borderline and malignant lesions [17].

A proportion of pregnant women with an ovarian cyst will require further imaging tests. In such cases, MRI is the test of choice. Contrary to ultrasonography, MRI is more operator-independent; moreover, it has excellent resolution for soft-tissue pathology, high sensitivity in identifying malignancy and negligible risks to the mother and fetus [18]. The use of gadolinium contrast medium should be avoided due to its teratogenic effect; actually, it is usually not required for the assessment of ovarian pathology [19]. Left lateral positioning should be considered to avoid caval compression by the gravid uterus in case of a prolonged stay in an MRI scan machine.

The use of CT for the assessment of ovarian cysts in pregnant women is not recommended; besides the well-established safety concerns about ionising radiation, CT actually performs poorly when compared to ultrasonography and therefore, it does not offer any clinical benefits [10].

1.4.2 Tumour Markers

Contrary to non-pregnant women, the use of serum tumour markers in patients with ovarian cysts during pregnancy is limited. The physiology of pregnancy alters baseline levels of some of these markers; the interpretation of abnormal results should be made with caution and always in conjunction with the results of imaging tests.

CA-125 is raised in about 80% of women with epithelial ovarian cancer, and it is the most frequently used serum tumour marker even though its specificity is low [13]. Its baseline levels increase in pregnancy; they peak in the first trimester with the upper limit of the normal CA-125 range reaching 112 U/mL between 11 and 14 weeks gestation and then decreasing as gestation advances [20]. Even though measuring CA-125 values per se will not discriminate between benign and malignant lesions in pregnancy, it may have some merits in suspicious or indeterminate ovarian cysts, as a significantly raised level may flag a potential malignancy and trigger further investigations. It may be measured as a reference point before and after treatment in women with known ovarian cancer, thus allowing physicians to monitor the response to treatment [6].

Other serum tumour markers used to monitor germ cell tumours include alpha-fetoprotein, human chorionic gonadotropin and lactate dehydrogenase. Unfortunately, the former two increase physiologically during pregnancy and therefore are of limited use. The latter is not affected by pregnancy, and its raised levels are a significant marker, commonly noted in dysgerminoma [6].

Finally, the glycoprotein HE4, which is a more sensitive and specific marker than CA-125 in differentiating between benign and malignant ovarian tumours, has lower baseline levels during pregnancy, hence limiting its potential use in pregnant women with ovarian lesions [6].

1.5 Management

Management of ovarian cysts diagnosed during pregnancy is challenging; physicians must address the individual needs of two patients, the mother and the fetus. Several factors need to be considered during decision-making: patient symptoms, gestational age and fetal well-being at the time of presentation, likelihood of malignancy or cyst accident, maternal and fetal risks associated with each management option, nature of surgical intervention and appropriate surgical approach. Each case needs to be assessed individually, ideally by a multidisciplinary team (MDT) comprising one or more obstetricians, gynaecologists, imaging specialists, paediatricians and midwives. In case a borderline or malignant ovarian lesion is suspected, then the case should also be referred to and managed by the gynaecology–oncology MDT including gynaecology oncologists, medical oncologists, radiologists, clinical nurse specialists and psychologists. This approach is likely to benefit the patient with a range of opinions and expertise collaborating in the management plan.

In general, the approach may include expectant management, ultrasound-guided fine needle aspiration or surgical management with the main determinants being patient symptoms and whether imaging findings are reassuring or raise any suspicions about malignancy.

1.5.1 Expectant Management

This is a safe approach in asymptomatic women with benign looking ovarian cysts without any suspicious imaging features; it is also supported by a recent evidence-based guideline commissioned by the British Society for Gynaecological Endoscopy (BSGE) and endorsed by the Royal College of Obstetricians and Gynaecologists (RCOG) [19]. The vast majority of cysts diagnosed in pregnancy are benign and actually, most of them are functional in nature. About 70% of them will resolve spontaneously by 16 weeks gestation and hence, no interventions are needed [4].

It has been suggested that cysts with benign features measuring more than 6 cm in size or those with a complex, albeit reassuring, ultrasound appearance should be followed up after four to six weeks [6, 10]. This is a reasonable practice but nevertheless, an experienced sonologist with expertise in women's imaging can, most of the time, offer reassurance about the scan findings and reduce the need for routine serial scans. Of course, certain types of benign ovarian cysts such as endometriomas should be followed up during pregnancy given the decidualisation-related diagnostic challenges.

When expectant management is favoured, women should be counselled about the risk of ovarian torsion and cyst rupture, and the plan should be reviewed if a patient becomes symptomatic and a cyst accident is suspected.

1.5.2 Ultrasound-Guided Fine Needle Aspiration

This option applies only to symptomatic women with simple benign ovarian cysts. It is a straight-forward outpatient procedure performed under local anaesthesia and it can provide immediate symptomatic relief, therefore reducing the need for admission and more invasive procedures. It is also included in the recent BSGE–RCOG guideline as an alternative option to surgery [19]. However, some authors have expressed concerns about high recurrence rates (33–40%), as well as the potential risk of intraperitoneal spillage of cancerous cells in the case of an undetected malignancy [5, 21].

1.5.3 Surgical Management

Surgery is usually reserved for patients with an acute abdomen due to a cyst accident and women with imaging findings suspicious of malignancy. It should also be considered in asymptomatic patients with large ovarian cysts (usually more than 10 cm, although there is no consensus in the literature about a cut-off limit) to prevent complications such as torsion, rupture or obstruction of labour [6].

Historically, the surgical approach included a laparotomy, nevertheless advances in minimal access surgery have now established laparoscopy as a safe and feasible approach during pregnancy [19]. A growing volume of literature evidence has demonstrated its superior outcomes in patients with benign disease and having addressed previous safety concerns, recent guidelines reflect the change in practice [19]. Laparoscopic surgery offers the same advantages to pregnant as to non-pregnant women. High quality studies have confirmed that laparoscopy is associated with improved visualisation of pelvic organs, reduced blood loss, less pain, reduced length of hospitalisation, faster recovery and a lower risk of uterine irritability compared to laparotomy, without an increase in adverse obstetric outcomes (miscarriage, preterm delivery or fetal growth restriction) [22, 23]. Patients mobilise more quickly following a laparoscopy, which is important given the hypercoagulable pregnancy status.

Previous concerns with regard to the impact of pneumoperitoneum and carbon dioxide on uteroplacental flow have now been discarded [24]. A study by Reedy et al. did not find any statistically significant differences in five fetal outcome variables (birth weight, gestational duration, growth restriction, infant survival and fetal malformations) in women with singleton pregnancies between 4–20 weeks of gestation undergoing laparoscopy versus laparotomy [25]. Most literature data as well as the BSUG–RCOG guidelines recommend an intra-abdominal operating pressure of 12 mmHg to minimise the risk of alterations to the feto-maternal perfusion, although visualisation may become more challenging [19, 24]. An operating pressure of 15 mmHg, however, has been used without adverse fetal or maternal outcomes [22, 26].

Another potential concern is related to the risk of inadvertent damage to the pregnant uterus with the Veress needle or the primary port during entry into the abdominal cavity. No randomised controlled trials have compared the safety of various laparoscopic entry points and techniques during pregnancy, therefore operating surgeons may utilise alternative options (e.g. open Hasson technique or direct gasless entry with optical trocar, entry at Palmer's point, supra-umbilical or sub-xiphoid point) according to their preference, fundal height and location of the ovarian cyst [19].

Despite its advantages, laparoscopic surgery during pregnancy can be technically challenging especially after the first trimester due to the enlarged pregnant uterus, absence of intra-uterine manipulation, relatively low intra-abdominal pressures and reduced intra-abdominal space. Therefore, it is recommended that that such procedures should be performed by experienced laparoscopic surgeons with advanced skills [19]. If malignancy is suspected pre- or intra-operatively, then a laparotomy should be considered to reduce the likelihood of cyst rupture and spillage of cancerous cells.

1.5.3.1 Elective versus Emergency Surgery

A recent systematic review and meta-analysis by Cagino et al. revealed that elective surgery during pregnancy is associated with a lower risk of preterm birth compared to emergency surgery [27]. As highlighted above, each case should be individually assessed within an MDT-based environment. Nevertheless, it seems that in the absence of any other robust data to guide counselling, elective surgery of asymptomatic, particularly large ovarian cysts should be considered to prevent complications and improve outcomes.

1.5.3.2 Cystectomy versus Oophorectomy

The decision on the nature of the surgical intervention (cystectomy versus oophorectomy or more radical surgery) depends on preoperative imaging and intra-operative surgical findings. Should there be no suspicion of malignancy, then a cystectomy is the approach of choice if feasible, with the aim to preserve as much healthy ovarian tissue as possible. Efforts should be made to avoid peritoneal spillage of cyst contents to prevent chemical peritonitis in the case of dermoid cysts and dissemination of malignant cells in the case of an undetected malignancy. The use of tissue removal bags or even in-bag dissection is encouraged. The corpus luteum should not be damaged if possible during surgical interventions in the first trimester. Drainage of benign looking ovarian cysts with or without concomitant cystectomy is an acceptable and safe alternative during pregnancy [19].

If a borderline or malignant ovarian lesion is suspected, then a two-stage approach could be considered especially in presumed early-stage disease; primary surgery during pregnancy may include a unilateral salpingo-oophorectomy and surgical staging (cytology, peritoneal biopsies, omentectomy and appendicectomy) with a completion staging surgery performed after delivery [28]. Of course, the gynaecology–oncology MDT will guide surgical planning of such cases.

1.5.3.3 When to Operate?

Historically, the second trimester was thought to be the ideal time to perform elective surgery in pregnancy, minimising the first and the third trimester risks of miscarriage and preterm birth, respectively. Nevertheless, this was not based on high quality evidence. A growing amount of literature data have demonstrated that laparoscopic surgery can be safely performed during all trimesters of pregnancy without any additional maternal and neonatal risks [25, 29]; recent evidence-based guidelines from the UK and US societies of endoscopic surgeons reflect this change in practice [19, 26].

Excision of an ovarian cyst at the time of a Caesarean section can be considered, especially if previous imaging has established that it is not a functional cyst or in the case of unexpected suspicious features. In general, management of such cases should be individualised and senior involvement should be sought in the case of an incidental finding of an ovarian cyst during a Caesarean section.

1.5.3.4 Obstetrical Considerations and Fetal Monitoring

Pre- and post-operative fetal heart monitoring is recommended to confirm fetal well-being. Contrary to past practice, routine intra-operative monitoring is no longer deemed necessary, as fetal heart and maternal uterine artery Doppler studies during laparoscopic surgery did not reveal any abnormalities [19, 24, 26].

Women undergoing surgery between 24 ± 0 and 35 ± 6 weeks gestation with a risk of preterm birth should be administrated antenatal corticosteroids for lung maturity; magnesium sulphate should also be used up 33 ± 6 weeks gestation for fetal neuroprotection as per the National Institute for Health and Care Excellence (NICE) guidelines [30].

Prophylactic administration of tocolytics has not been found to improve outcomes and hence, it is not routinely recommended; of course, should there be signs of preterm birth, this can be considered [19, 26].

1.6 Post-Natal Follow-Up

Post-natal ultrasound evaluation of persistent ovarian cysts, usually six weeks postpartum, is a reasonable approach. At this stage, patients will be able to undergo elective surgery if deemed necessary [10].

1.7 Conclusion

Since ultrasonography was established as an integral part of antenatal care, the incidence of diagnosis of ovarian cysts in pregnant women has increased. The vast majority of them are functional in nature; such cysts can be safely managed expectantly. The main objective of assessment and management is to exclude possible acute cyst accidents, triage and fast-track cysts with suspicious features and optimise maternal and fetal outcomes; however, this can often be challenging due to the pregnant state of patients masking pathology or confounding symptoms. Shared decision-making within an MDT-based environment is encouraged.

Clinical Governance Issues

- Most ovarian cysts encountered in pregnancy are functional in nature and will resolve spontaneously by 16 weeks gestation
- Accurate characterisation of the nature of the cysts is essential. Approximately 1–5% and 1–2% of them will represent a malignant (most commonly germ cell, sex cord stromal and epithelial tumours) and a borderline lesion (predominantly serous and mucinous borderline tumours), respectively
- The possibility of a cyst accident (e.g. ovarian torsion, cyst rupture and haemorrhage) should always be considered in pregnant women presenting with lower abdominal pain
- About 10–20% of all cases of ovarian torsion occur during pregnancy, usually between 10–17 weeks gestation
- Although ovarian torsion has distinct ultrasound features, it still remains a clinical diagnosis. In the absence of convincing imaging features, physicians should strongly consider proceeding to surgical intervention should the clinical findings be highly suspicious of ovarian torsion
- Ultrasonography is the first-line imaging modality in pregnant women with an ovarian cyst
- The IOTA group's 'simple descriptors' and 'simple rules' have high sensitivity and specificity in differentiating between benign and malignant ovarian cysts
- Endometriomas may undergo major sonographic changes during pregnancy (decidualisation) and mimic malignancy
- Physiology of pregnancy alters baseline levels of most tumour markers, hence their role during pregnancy is limited
- MRI can be a useful diagnostic tool should ultrasonography be inconclusive, as it has excellent resolution for soft-tissue pathology, high sensitivity in identifying malignancy and negligible risks to mother and fetus

- Pregnant women with an ovarian cyst should be managed within an MDT-based environment
- Expectant management is a safe option in asymptomatic women with benign looking ovarian cysts
- Ultrasound-guided fine needle aspiration is a reasonable alternative in symptomatic women with simple benign ovarian cysts despite the high recurrence rates
- Surgery should be considered in patients with acute abdomen, women with suspected malignancy and possibly in asymptomatic patients with large ovarian cysts to prevent future complications
- Laparoscopic surgery in all trimesters of pregnancy is feasible and safe both for the mother and fetus. It should be performed by experienced surgeons with advanced laparoscopic skills especially at advanced gestational age

References

1 N. Schwartz, I. E. Timor-Tritsch and E. Wang. Adnexal masses in pregnancy. *Clinical Obstetrics and Gynecology,* **52** (2009), 570–85.

2 K. E. Webb, K. Sakhel, S. P. Chauhan and A. Z. Abuhamad. Adnexal mass during pregnancy: A review. *American Journal of Perinatology,* **32** (2015), 1010–16.

3 K. M. Schmeler, W. W. Mayo-Smith, J. F. Peipert, et al. Adnexal masses in pregnancy: Surgery compared with observation. *Obstetrics and Gynecology,* **105** (2005), 1098–103.

4 G. Condous, A. Khalid, E. Okaro and T. Bourne. Should we be examining the ovaries in pregnancy? Prevalence and natural history of adnexal pathology detected at first-trimester sonography. *Ultrasound in Obstetrics & Gynecology: The Official Journal of the International Society of Ultrasound in Obstetrics and Gynecology,* **24** (2004), 62–6.

5 C. Bottomley and T. Bourne. Diagnosis and management of ovarian cyst accidents. *Best Practice & Research Clinical Obstetrics & Gynaecology,* **23** (2009), 711–24.

6 A. O. Alalade and H. Maraj. Management of adnexal masses in pregnancy. *Obstetrician & Gynaecologist,* **19** (2017), 317–25.

7 C. Huang, M. K. Hong and D. C. Ding. A review of ovary torsion. *Ci ji yi xue za zhi = Tzu-chi Medical Journal,* **29** (2017), 143–7.

8 C. F. Yen, S. L. Lin, W. Murk, et al. Risk analysis of torsion and malignancy for adnexal masses during pregnancy. *Fertility and Sterility,* **91** (2009), 1895–902.

9 M. Graif and Y. Itzchak. Sonographic evaluation of ovarian torsion in childhood and adolescence. *American Journal of Roentgenology,* **150** (1988), 647–9.

10 S. Senarath, A. Ades and P. Nanayakkara. Ovarian cysts in pregnancy: A narrative review. *Journal of Obstetrics and Gynaecology: The Journal of the Institute of Obstetrics and Gynaecology,* **41** (2021), 169–75.

11 R. Eskander, M. Berman and L. Keder. Practice Bulletin No. 174: Evaluation and management of adnexal masses. *Obstetrics and Gynecology,* **128** (2016), e210–e26.

12 A. Sokalska, D. Timmerman, A. C. Testa, et al. Diagnostic accuracy of transvaginal ultrasound examination for assigning a specific diagnosis to adnexal masses. *Ultrasound in Obstetrics & Gynecology: The Official Journal of the International Society of Ultrasound in Obstetrics and Gynecology,* **34** (2009), 462–70.

13 P. Kaloo, K. Louden, S. Khazali and D. Hoy. *RCOG/BSGE National Green Top Guidelines No: 62, 'Management of Suspected Ovarian Masses in Premenopausal Women'.* (November 2011).

14 J. Yazbek, S. K. Raju, J. Ben-Nagi, et al. Effect of quality of gynaecological ultrasonography on management of patients with suspected ovarian cancer: A randomised controlled trial. *Lancet Oncology,* **9** (2008), 124–31.

15 D. Timmerman, A. C. Testa, T. Bourne, et al. Simple ultrasound-based rules for the diagnosis of ovarian cancer. *Ultrasound in Obstetrics & Gynecology: The Official Journal of the International Society of Ultrasound in Obstetrics and Gynecology,* **31** (2008), 681–90.

16 L. Ameye, D. Timmerman, L. Valentin, et al. Clinically oriented three-step strategy for assessment of adnexal pathology. *Ultrasound in Obstetrics & Gynecology: The Official Journal of the International Society of Ultrasound in Obstetrics and Gynecology,* **40** (2012), 582–91.

17 K. Pateman, F. Moro, D. Mavrelos, et al. Natural history of ovarian endometrioma in pregnancy. *BMC Women's Health,* **14** (2014), 128.

18 S. Adusumilli, H. K. Hussain, E. M. Caoili, et al. MRI of sonographically indeterminate adnexal masses. *American Journal of Roentgenology,* **187** (2006), 732–40.

19 E. Ball, N. Waters, N. Cooper, et al. Evidence-based guideline on laparoscopy in pregnancy: Commissioned by the British Society for Gynaecological Endoscopy (BSGE), endorsed by the Royal College of Obstetricians & Gynaecologists (RCOG). *Facts, Views & Vision in ObGyn,* **11** (2019), 5–25.

20 N. Aslam, C. Ong, B. Woelfer, K. Nicolaides and D. Jurkovic. Serum CA125 at 11–14 weeks of gestation in women with morphologically normal ovaries. *BJOG: An International Journal of Obstetrics and Gynaecology,* **107** (2000), 689–90.

21 L. Guariglia, M. Conte, P. Are and P. Rosati. Ultrasound-guided fine needle aspiration of ovarian cysts during pregnancy. *European Journal of Obstetrics, Gynecology, and Reproductive Biology,* **82** (1999), 5–9.

22 L. Chen, J. Ding and K. Hua. Comparative analysis of laparoscopy versus laparotomy in the management of ovarian cyst during pregnancy. *Journal of Obstetrics and Gynaecology Research,* **40** (2014), 763–9.

23 Y. X. Liu, Y. Zhang, J. F. Huang and L. Wang. Meta-analysis comparing the safety of laparoscopic and open surgical approaches for suspected adnexal mass during the second trimester. *International Journal of Gynaecology and Obstetrics: The Official Organ of the International Federation of Gynaecology and Obstetrics,* **136** (2017), 272–9.

24 M. Candiani, S. Maddalena, M. Barbieri, et al. Adnexal masses in pregnancy: Fetomaternal blood flow indices during laparoscopic surgery. *Journal of Minimally Invasive Gynecology,* **19** (2012), 443–7.

25 M. B. Reedy, B. Källén and T. J. Kuehl. Laparoscopy during pregnancy: A study of five fetal outcome parameters with use of the Swedish Health Registry. *American Journal of Obstetrics and Gynecology,* **177** (1997), 673–9.

26 J. P. Pearl, R. R. Price, A. E. Tonkin, W. S. Richardson and D. Stefanidis. SAGES guidelines for the use of laparoscopy during pregnancy. *Surgical Endoscopy,* **31** (2017), 3767–82.

27 K. Cagino, X. Li, C. Thomas, et al. Surgical management of adnexal masses in pregnancy: A systematic review and meta-analysis. *Journal of Minimally Invasive Gynecology,* **28** (2021), 1171–82.

28 A. Mukhopadhyay, A. Shinde and R. Naik. Ovarian cysts and cancer in pregnancy. *Best Practice & Research Clinical Obstetrics & Gynaecology,* **33** (2016), 58–72.

29 E. Weiner, Y. Mizrachi, R. Keidar, et al. Laparoscopic surgery performed in advanced pregnancy compared to early pregnancy. *Archives of Gynecology and Obstetrics,* **292** (2015), 1063–8.

30 National Collaborating Centre for Women's and Children's Health. *Preterm Labour and Birth.* (London: National Institute for Health and Care Excellence, 2015).

Fibroids in Pregnancy

T. Justin Clark, Lina Antoun

Chapter

2

2.1 Introduction

Fibroids (leiomyomas) are the most common benign tumour in women with a prevalence of 20–50% in women older than 30 years. Fibroids have a higher prevalence in African American women (60%), and are less common in white women (40%) [1]. The incidence of fibroids during pregnancy is increasing due to advanced maternal age with a prevalence of 10.7% in the first trimester [1, 2]. Most pregnant women with fibroids do not have any problems during pregnancy, whereas 10–30% of fibroids affect pregnancy in the intrapartum period and during delivery [3]. Complications during pregnancy depend on the size and location of the fibroids. Large submucosal or multiple fibroids in addition to cervical and retro-placental fibroids have a greater risk of complication including the risk of post-partum haemorrhage (PPH), which is the second most common cause of direct maternal death [4]. Additional risks of fibroids include peripartum hysterectomy, malpresentation, placental abruption, placenta praevia, preterm labour, preterm premature rupture of membranes (PPROM) and increasing Caesarean section rates [5, 6]. Currently, there is no standardised guideline in the UK to manage pregnant women with fibroids. The consensus is to individualise the care for these women based on the effect of the fibroid on the course of pregnancy, delivery plans and the woman's desire for fertility.

2.2 Types of Fibroids

The International Federation of Gynaecology and Obstetrics' (FIGO) classification of fibroids, which incorporates the original European Society of Gynaecological Endoscopy (ESGE) classification for submucous fibroids, is the most widely adopted (Table 2.1) [7, 8].

Fibroids can be located in the uterine body, broad ligament or cervix. Fibroids within the uterine body are either submucosal, intramural or subserosal [7, 8]. Broad ligament fibroids are located in the peritoneal folds of the broad ligaments and can lead to displacement of the uterus. Cervical fibroids can obstruct fetal head engagement and lead to malpresentation [3]. Both broad ligament and cervical fibroids can pose a challenge during a Caesarean section [2].

2.3 The Effect of Pregnancy on Fibroids

Fibroids are hormone-dependent lesions. In addition to placental oestrogens and progesterone, there are other factors that may affect fibroid blood supply and growth rate during pregnancy. Fibroids can shrink, increase in size or remain the same antenatally [9, 10]. One-third of fibroids increase in size in the first trimester [11] and therefore, the

Table 2.1 FIGO and ESGE classification of uterine fibroids

ESGE	Fibroid type	FIGO	Fibroid type	Location
No myometrial involvement – pedunculated	0	Submucosal	0	Pedunculated in the cavity
<50% myometrial involvement	1		1	<50% intramural
			2	≥50% intramural
		Intramural	3	Contacts endometrium, 100% intramural
			4	100% intramural
		Subserosal	5	Subserous and ≥50% intramural
≥50% myometrial involvement	2		6	Subserous and <50% intramural
		Pedunculated	7	Subserous pedunculated
		Other	8	Cervical/parasitic
		Hybrid leiomyoma	2–5	Submucous and subserous, each with less than half the diameter in the endometrial and peritoneal cavities

location and size of the fibroids should be assessed from the first trimester. Cervical fibroids may move upwards as the pregnancy advances, after the development of the lower uterine segment [11].

2.4 The Effect of Fibroids on the Pregnancy

Overall, 10–40% of women with fibroids will develop maternal and fetal complications during pregnancy [12]. Complications are more common in larger fibroids (>200 cm^3 in volume or >5 cm in diameter) [12].

2.4.1 Multiple Large Fibroids in the Anterior Wall and Lower Segment
2.4.1.1 Maternal Complications

Subfertility is present in 5–10% of women with fibroids with two-thirds of these women conceiving following abdominal myomectomy [13].

In pregnancy, abdominal pain is the most common complication of fibroids. Pain is mostly seen in fibroids measuring >5 cm in diameter during the second and third trimesters [12, 14]. The pain is often secondary to red degeneration of the fibroid due to tissue anoxia and necrosis. This could be the result of a rapidly growing fibroid in pregnancy or growth of a gravid uterus, which affects the blood supply to the fibroid leading to ischaemia [12]. A less common reason for fibroid pain in pregnancy is a torsion of a pedunculated fibroid [12]. Other symptoms like urinary obstruction, increasing urinary frequency and bowel disturbance can be the result of a large fibroid pressing on the bowel, the bladder and the ureters [12, 13].

Submucosal fibroids can lead to subfertility, bleeding and miscarriage [15]. Uterine fibroids increase the risk of bleeding in pregnancy [16]. The presence of a large fibroid in pregnancy doubles the risk of placenta praevia [14, 15]. Submucosal or large fibroids which are located close to the placental site can affect the blood flow to the placenta and increase the risk of placental abruption [6, 13].

During delivery, lower segment fibroids can obstruct the delivery leading to higher Caesarean section rates and retained placental tissues [2, 12]. Following delivery, fibroids can impact on uterine contractibility leading to PPH [17].

2.4.1.2 Fetal Complications

Fibroids are associated with a 14% risk of miscarriage in the first trimester compared to an 8% risk of miscarriage in women without fibroids [18]. This could be the result of a poor blood supply to the fetus due the physical presence of a fibroid(s) [19, 20]. The risk of miscarriage increases with large or multiple fibroids [19]. Fibroids present in the uterine body have a higher rate of miscarriage compared to lower segment fibroids [19]. Large submucosal fibroids can cause a compression and distortion in the endometrial cavity leading to intra-uterine fetal growth restriction and fetal structural anomalies [20]. These anomalies include dolichocephaly (lateral compression of the fetal skull), limb reduction defects and torticollis (abnormal twisting of the neck) [21, 22].

Multiple large fibroids (greater than 5 cm in diameter), and lower segment fibroids are risk factors for fetal malpresentation [16, 19, 23]. Another obstetric complication with fibroids is preterm labour, which is significantly higher in those with fibroids compared to women without fibroids (16.1% compared to 8.7%) [15].

2.4.2 Large Cervical Fibroids

Women with large cervical fibroids or fibroids near the placental site should be booked under consultant-led care to discuss the implications of the fibroids in pregnancy and individualise a management plan. Cervical fibroids can be classified as intracervical (located within the cervix) or extracervical (surrounding the cervical canal and displacing the uterus) [24].

Central cervical fibroids surrounding the cervical canal can obstruct labour. The mode of delivery for these women should be by an elective Caesarean section, with conservative management of the fibroids during the Caesarean section.

Large cervical fibroids (>5 cm in diameter) can cause pain and pressure symptoms especially in the second and third trimesters [25]. There is also a risk of spontaneous rupture of membranes (SROM) and cord prolapse with large cervical fibroids [26].

2.4.2.1 Cervical Fibroid Polyps in the Vagina

Pedunculated cervical fibroids in the vagina can originate from the uterine cavity or endocervical canal [12, 13, 26]. These can increase in size in pregnancy and lead to recurrent vaginal bleeding [25]. These patients can be managed conservatively during pregnancy. Vaginal myomectomy can be an option in certain cases especially with recurrent heavy vaginal bleeding necessitating blood transfusion [25].

2.5 Antenatal Management of Women with Fibroids

Optimisation of anaemia prior to delivery is essential to reduce complications from PPH and the need for blood transfusion [27]. Measuring symphysial fundal height in not reliable in women with multiple or large fibroids (>5 cm in diameter). These women are advised to undergo serial growth scans from 28 weeks to identify intra-uterine growth restricted babies and detect fetal malpresentation in the third trimester of pregnancy [28].

Ultrasound scan surveillance (USS) helps to identify rapidly growing fibroids, which allows early intervention in the unusual case of malignancy. In case of difficulty characterising the fibroids using USS, MRI may provide further information, and differentiate between atypical leiomyomas and uterine sarcomas [29]. MRI can be performed safely in pregnancy [30]. Abdominal pain in pregnant women with fibroids can be the result of red degeneration, pressure symptoms or torsion of pedunculated fibroids, especially in the second and third trimesters [3, 5, 9]. It is important to exclude other causes of abdominal pain including preterm labour. Physical examination and USS are useful in pregnant women with known fibroids and who present with acute pain [6].

Paracetamol and opioid analgesics such as morphine are safe in pregnancy. NSAIDS are effective in fibroid pain but they need to be used with caution in the third trimester because of the risk of premature closure of the ductus arteriosus, leading to fetal pulmonary hypertension [31]. Uterine fibroids are not a contraindication to external cephalic version (ECV) [32] for women with malpresentation in the absence of significant cervical fibroid(s).

Antenatal myomectomy may rarely be required for recurrent bleeding or severe pain from a degenerating fibroid, especially a rapidly enlarging fibroid or a pedunculated, torted fibroid. Antenatal myomectomy is considered to be safer during the first and second trimesters [33, 34]. A study comparing the outcome in women with fibroids who underwent antepartum myomectomy with women who did not [34], demonstrated that antepartum myomectomy is beneficial in improving reproductive and pregnancy outcomes when performed early in selected patients. There was in an increase the rate of Caesarean section in women who underwent antepartum myomectomy, in addition to prolonged hospital stays post-operatively, but no increased risk of peripartum hysterectomy [33]. Antenatal myomectomy is not routine practice in the UK, therefore, pregnant women who require antepartum myomectomy should be transferred to centres with expertise in performing such procedures.

2.6 Counselling about the Risks and Impact of Fibroids on Mode of Delivery

2.6.1 Vaginal Delivery

Pregnant women with fibroids are considered to be high risk, and are advised to deliver in units with facilities for cell salvage and blood transfusion in view of the increased risk of PPH and Caesarean hysterectomy [12, 18].

Vaginal delivery should not be attempted in women with cervical fibroids, or large lower segment fibroids causing fetal malpresentation or obstructing labour [25].

Women who are deemed suitable for a vaginal delivery and particularly women following previous myomectomy will need intravenous access and continuous fetal heart monitoring during labour in order to detect early uterine rupture [35].

Pregnant women with fibroids are advised to have active management of the third stage of labour and uterotonics following delivery to reduce the risk of PPH [36].

Balloon tamponade and uterine packing can be attempted in the case of ongoing PPH [36], however, large submucosal fibroids might affect the placement of the balloon in the uterine cavity. In the case of major obstetric haemorrhage (>1000 ml blood loss), the Royal College of Obstetrics and Gynaecology (RCOG) has set specific recommendations [36] to help manage such situations including the advice to deliver in high-risk consultant-led units where the facilities for cell salvage and interventional radiology can be utilised. Uterine B-Lynch suture, internal iliac artery ligation, uterine artery ligation and peripartum hysterectomy are all part of the management protocol for PPH. Tranexamic acid can also be given in order to help manage PPH in these cases [36].

2.6.2 Caesarean Section

Elective Caesarean section is advised in the case of central cervical fibroids and lower segment fibroids obstructing labour or leading to malpresentation [26]. The Caesarean section may be challenging in the presence of cervical fibroids, large lower segment fibroids and extensive adhesions from previous myomectomies because of difficulty accessing the lower uterine segment of the uterus to facilitate safe delivery [37].

In these situations, a classical uterine incision should be considered, trying to avoid the fibroid to prevent severe, major PPH. Broad ligament fibroids can deviate the uterus laterally, distorting the anatomy and therefore, it is very important to identify anatomical structures in these cases before proceeding with the Caesarean section to reduce the risk of injury [12, 14].

Women with large or cervical fibroids should be consented for a Caesarean section hysterectomy in the case of uncontrolled PPH, and admission to intensive care.

A subumbilical midline incision can be considered in women who have a history of previous anterior myomectomy and where significant pelvic adhesions are anticipated [38].

The bladder may also be higher than expected in patients with a history of previous myomectomy, therefore, care must be taken when reflecting the bladder down during the Caesarean section in such cases [38]. The uterine arteries can be ligated immediately following the Caesarean section to reduce blood loss and subsequently, the risk of peripartum hysterectomy [39]. It is imperative to identify the ureters in women with broad ligament fibroids requiring peripartum hysterectomy in order to reduce the risk of ureteric injury [40]. Tranexamic acid can be given during Caesarean section in the presence of a fibroid uterus to reduce the risk of PPH [36].

Myomectomy can be performed at the time of the Caesarean section in order to facilitate safe delivery of the baby or if the fibroids are interfering with the closure of the uterine incision [41]. Caesarean section myomectomy was not found to significantly affect blood loss or post-operative complications; however, it was found to increase the risk of placenta praevia in future pregnancies [28, 41]. Spontaneous conception was as high as 79% following a Caesarean myomectomy compared to 38.6–55.9% following a later interval myomectomy [42].

2.7 Delivery with History of Previous Myomectomy

Pregnant women with previous myomectomy could be managed similarly to those attempting vaginal birth with previous Caesarean section. Elective Caesarean section should be considered if there is a history of previous myomectomy to reduce the risk of uterine rupture in case of the following [42]:

1. Breach in the endometrial cavity
2. Large defect
3. Laparoscopic myomectomy for intramural or submucosal fibroids

The risk of uterine rupture following laparoscopic myomectomy was found to be 1.2% [43, 44], compared to a lower risk of 0.4% following abdominal myomectomy [45]. The higher risk of uterine rupture following laparoscopic myomectomy may be a result of the excessive use of diathermy during the procedure and the difficulty in the multi-layer closure of the myometrium during laparoscopy [28]. There is no robust evidence to advise on the mode of delivery following myomectomy. A meta-analysis [36] has quoted a vaginal delivery success rate of 90% following open and laparoscopic myomectomy. Uterine rupture cases following myomectomy are more common in the third trimester and during labour [42]. The time interval between the delivery and the myomectomy may be a relevant factor that affects the risk [43].

MRI findings suggest that the endometrium should be fully healed three months following open myomectomy [44]. For laparoscopic myomectomy, the recommendation is at least a six-month interval between the surgery and subsequent pregnancies [46]. Due to concerns about uterine rupture, women are advised to deliver at 37–38 weeks of gestation [36, 44].

2.8 Post-Natal Management of Women with Fibroids

Fibroids shrink in size in >70% of women by six months post-natally [46]. Pyomyoma is a rare life-threatening complication of fibroids in the post-partum period resulting from necrosis, secondary infection and infarction of the fibroids [47]. Pyomyoma can manifest with abdominal pain and sepsis without any obvious source of infection in the presence of a leiomyoma [47]. Pedunculated submucosal fibroids are more prone to necrosis due to the poor blood supply through the stalk [47]. Computed tomography-guided drainage is possible. The diagnosis is usually confirmed by exploratory laparotomy. Surgical intervention by laparotomy and myomectomy or hysterectomy combined with appropriate antibiotic treatment can improve the clinical prognosis [47].

Clinical Governance Issues

- Thorough counselling regarding the risk of uterine rupture during labour should be undertaken prior to attempting vaginal delivery in women with a history of previous myomectomy
- An elective Caesarean section is advisable in women who have undergone a previous myomectomy if there has been a breach in the endometrial cavity, there has been a

significant myometrial defect from the removal of large or multiple intramural fibroids or after laparoscopic myomectomy for large intramural or submucosal fibroids
- Myomectomy should only be performed during Caesarean section if the delivery of the baby is not feasible without myomectomy

References

1 D. D. Baird, D. B. Dunson, M. C. Hill, et al. High cumulative incidence of uterine leiomyoma in black and white women: Ultrasound evidence. *American Journal of Obstetrics and Gynecology*, **188** (2003), 100–7.

2 D. H. Kwon, J. E. Song, K. R. Yoon, et al. The safety of caesarean myomectomy in women with large myomas. *Obstetrics and Gynecology Science*, **57** (2014), 367–72.

3 M. Deveer, R, Deveer, Y. Engin-Ustun, et al. Comparison of pregnancy outcomes in different localizations of uterine fibroids. *Clinical and Experimental Obstetrics and Gynecology*, **39** (2012), 516–18.

4 M. Knight, D. Tuffnell, S. Kenyon, et al. *Saving lives improving mothers' care-surveillance of maternal deaths in the UK2011–13 and lessons learned to inform maternity care from the UK and Ireland Confidential Enquiries into Maternal Deaths and Morbidity 2009–13.* (Oxford: MBRRACE-UK, 2015). www.npeu.ox.ac.uk/mbrrace-uk/presentations/saving-lives-improving-mothers-care

5 G. D. Coronado, L. M. Marshall and S. M. Schwartz. Complications in pregnancy, labor, and delivery with uterine leiomyomas: A population-based study. *Obstetrics & Gynecology*, **95** (2000), 764–69.

6 C. Exacoustos and P. Rosati. Ultrasound diagnosis of uterine myomas and complications in pregnancy. *Obstetrics & Gynecology*, **82** (1993), 97–101.

7 M. G. Munro, H. O. Critchley, M. S. Broder, et al. FIGO working group on menstrual disorders. FIGO classification system (PALM-COEIN) for causes of abnormal uterine bleeding in nongravid women of reproductive age. *International Journal of Gynaecology & Obstetrics*, **113** (2011), 3–13.

8 K. Wamsteker, M. H. Emanuel and J. H. de Kruif. Transcervical hysteroscopic resection of submucous fibroids for abnormal uterine bleeding: Results regarding the degree of intramural extension. *Obstetrics & Gynecology*, **82** (1993), 736–40.

9 R. Neiger, J. D. Sonek, C. S. Croom, et al. Pregnancy-related changes in the size of uterine leiomyomas. *Journal of Reproductive Medicine*, **51** (2006), 671–4.

10 A. O. Hammoud, R. Asaad, J. Berman, et al. Volume change of uterine myomas during pregnancy: Do myomas really grow? *Journal of Minimally Invasive Gynecology*, **13** (2006), 386–90.

11 P. Rosati, C. Exacoustos and S. Mancuso. Longitudinal evaluation of uterine myoma growth during pregnancy. A sonographic study. *Journal of Ultrasound in Medicine*, **11** (1992), 511–15.

12 V. L. Katz, D. J. Dotters and W. Droegemueller. Complications of uterine leiomyomas in pregnancy. *Obstetrics & Gynecology*, **73** (1989), 593–6.

13 Y. Khalaf and S. K. Sunkara. The patient with fibroids. In: N. Macklon, ed., *IVF in the Medically Complicated Patient: A Guide to Management* (Boca Raton: CRC Press, 2014), pp. 129–35.

14 C. A. Burton, D. A. Grimes and C. M. March. Surgical management of leiomyomata during pregnancy. *Obstetrics & Gynecology*, **74** (1989), 707–9.

15 P. C. Klatsky, N. D. Tran, A. B. Caughey, et al. Fibroids and reproductive

outcomes: A systematic literature review from conception to delivery. *American Journal of Obstetrics and Gynecology*, **198** (2008), 357–66.

16 J. P. Rice, H. H. Kay and B. S. Mahony. The clinical significance of uterine leiomyomas in pregnancy. *American Journal of Obstetrics and Gynecology*, **160** (1989), 1212–16.

17 J. Szamatowicz, T. Laudanski, B. Bulkszas, et al. Fibromyomas and uterine contractions. *Acta Obstetrica et Gynecologia Scandinavica*, **76** (1997), 973–6.

18 C. B. Benson, J. S. Chow, W. Chang-Lee, et al. Outcome of pregnancies in women with uterine leiomyomas identified by sonography in the first trimester. *Journal of Clinical Ultrasound*, **29** (2001), 261–4.

19 A. S. Lev-Toaff, B. G. Coleman, P. H. Arger, et al. Leiomyomas in pregnancy: Sonographic study. *Radiology*, **164** (1987), 375–80.

20 H. J. Lee, E. R. Norwitz and J. Shaw. Contemporary management of fibroids in pregnancy. *Reviews in Obstetrics and Gynecology*, **3** (2010), 20–7.

21 J. M. Graham Jr, M. E. Miller, M. J. Stephan, et al. Limb reduction anomalies and early in utero limb compression. *The Journal of Pediatrics*, **96** (1980), 1052–6.

22 J. Chuang, H. W. Tsai and J. L. Hwang. Fetal compression syndrome caused by myoma in pregnancy: A case report. *Acta Obstetrica et Gynecologia Scandinavica*, **80** (2001), 472–3.

23 P. Vergani, A. Locatelli, A. Ghidini, et al. Large uterine leiomyomata and risk of Cesarean delivery. *Obstetrics & Gynecology*, **109** (2007), 410–14

24 F. Ferrari, S. Forte, G. Valenti, et al. Current treatment options for cervical leiomyomas: A systematic review of literature. *Medicina (Kaunas)*, **57** (2021), 92.

25 R. Keriakos and M. Maher. Management of cervical fibroid during the reproductive period. *Case Reports in Obstetrics and Gynecology*, (2013), doi:10.1155/2013/

984030. Epub 2013 Sep 15. PMID: 24109537.

26 M. M. Abitbol and R. L. Madison. Cervical fibroids complicating pregnancy. *Obstetrics & Gynecology*, **12** (1958), 397–98.

27 G. Mollica, L. Pittini, E. Minganti, et al. Elective uterine myomectomy in pregnant women. *Clinical and Experimental Obstetrics & Gynecology*, **23** (1996), 168–72.

28 Royal College of Obstetricians and Gynaecologists. *The Investigation and Management of the Small-for-Gestational-Age Fetus. Green-top Guideline No. 31.* (London: RCOG, 2014). www.rcog.org .uk/en/guidelines-research-services/ guidelines/gtg31/

29 A. Suzuki, M. Aoki, C. Miyagawa, et al. Differential diagnosis of uterine leiomyoma and uterine sarcoma using magnetic resonance images: A literature review. *Healthcare (Basel)*, **7** (2019), 158.

30 B. M. Mervak, E. Altun, K. A. McGinty, et al. MRI in pregnancy: Indications and practical considerations. *Journal of Magnetic Resonance Imaging*, **49** (2019), 621–31.

31 H. J. Lee, E. R. Norwitz and J. Shaw. Contemporary management of fibroids in pregnancy. *Reviews in Obstetrics and Gynecology*, **3** (2010), 20–7.

32 L. W. M. Impey, D. J. Murphy, M, Griffiths, et al. On behalf of the Royal College of Obstetricians and Gynaecologists. External cephalic version and reducing the incidence of term breech presentation. *British Journal of Obstetrics and Gynaecology*, **124** (2017), e178–92.

33 S. De Carolis, G. Fatigante, S. Ferrazzani, et al. Uterine myomectomy in pregnant women. *Fetal Diagnosis and Therapy*, **16** (2001),116–19.

34 G. Mollica, L. Pittini, E. Minganti, G. Perri and F. Pansini. Elective uterine myomectomy in pregnant women. *Clinical and Experimental Obstetrics & Gynecology*, **23** (1996),168–72.

35 J. Claeys, I. Hellendoorn, T. Hamerlynck, et al. The risk of uterine rupture after myomectomy: A systematic review of the literature and meta-analysis. *Gynecological Surgery,* **11** (2014), 197.

36 E. Mavrides, S. Allard, E. Chandraharan, et al. Prevention and management of postpartum haemorrhage: Green-top guideline No. 52. *British Journal of Obstetrics and Gynaecology,* **124** (2017), e106–149. doi:10.1111/1471-0528.14178. Epub 2016 Dec 16.

37 H. Li, J. Du, L. Jin, et al. Myomectomy during Cesarean section. *Acta Obstetrica et Gynecologia Scandinavica,* **88** (2009),183–6.

38 P. Seinera, R. Arisio, A. Decko, et al. Laparoscopic myomectomy: Indications, surgical technique and complications. *Human Reproduction,* **12** (1997), 1927–30.

39 W. M. Liu, P. H. Wang, W. L. Tang, et al. Uterine artery ligation for treatment of pregnant women with uterine leiomyomas who are undergoing Cesarean section. *Fertility and Sterility,* **86** (2006), 423–8.

40 T. Lopes, N. Spirtos, R. Naik and J. Monaghan. Uterine fibroids. In: *Bonney's Gynaecological Surgery,* 11th ed. (Chichester: Blackwell, 2010), pp. 87–94.

41 D. Song, W. Zhang, M. C. Chames, et al. Myomectomy during Caesarean delivery. *International Journal of Gynecology & Obstetrics,* **121** (2013), 208–13.

42 E. Y. Kwawukume. Caesarean myomectomy. *African Journal of Reproductive Health,* **6** (2002), 38–43.

43 C. Gyamfi-Bannerman, S. Gilbert, M. B. Landon, et al. Risk of uterine rupture and placenta accreta with prior uterine surgery outside of the lower segment. *Obstetrics & Gynecology,* **120** (2012), 1332–7.

44 S. Tsuji, K. Takahashi, I. Imaoka, et al. MRI evaluation of the uterine structure after myomectomy. *Gynecological and Obstetric Investigation,* **61** (2006), 106–10.

45 T. S. Bernardi, M. P. Radosa, A. Weisheit, et al. Laparoscopic myomectomy: A 6-year follow-up single-center cohort analysis of fertility and obstetric outcome measures. *Archives of Gynecology and Obstetrics,* **290** (2014), 87–91.

46 Society of Obstetricians and Gynaecologists of Canada. The management of uterine leiomyomas. SOGC clinical practice guideline 318. *Journal of Obstetrics and Gynaecology Canada,* **37** (2015), 157–78.

47 C. Del Borgo, F. Maneschi, V. Belvisi, et al. Postpartum fever in the presence of a fibroid: Sphingomonas paucimobilis sepsis associated with pyomyoma. *BMC Infectious Diseases,* **13** (2013), 574.

Chapter 3

Cervical Abnormalities in Pregnancy

Parveen Abedin, Lina Antoun

3.1 Introduction

Cervical intra-epithelial neoplasia (CIN) is a precancerous lesion common in women of reproductive age [1].

The incidence of invasive cervical cancer has decreased markedly in the last 30 years owing to far-reaching screening programmes that have led to the early diagnosis and treatment of CIN amongst asymptomatic women [2]. Effective treatment of high-grade lesions is important to prevent cervical cancer. However, only a small proportion of low-grade lesions progress to high-grade lesions or invasive cancer, and approximately 50% regress back to normal in two years [3, 4].

During pregnancy, the regression, persistence and progression rate of high-grade CIN are 40%, 59% and 1%, respectively; hence, the case can be made for conservative management of CIN2/3 [5].

Furthermore, during pregnancy, approximately 2–7 women in 100 will experience abnormal cervical cytological findings and 1.3–2.7% will be affected by different degrees of CIN [5].

In the United Kingdom, most of these women will either have no procedure (and be discharged) or have a punch biopsy sample taken at their first colposcopy appointment to confirm the presence or absence of disease, whereas others (particularly those with high-grade cytological abnormalities) may be offered excisional treatment at the first visit [6].

Several techniques have been used in the treatment of pre-invasive lesions, such as cold-knife conisation, laser ablation, laser conisation and a loop electrosurgical excision procedure (LEEP), also known as large loop excision of the transformation zone (LLETZ) [7]. The latter technique has become the standard treatment for women affected by precancerous cervical lesions, mainly based on its low rate of morbidity, the possibility of assessing completeness of excision on histology and the ability to combine diagnosis and therapy in an outpatient clinic [8].

3.1.1 LLETZ and Obstetric Outcomes

The incidence of CIN peaks among women during their reproductive age; consequently, any possible effect of its treatment on future childbearing should be considered carefully [9]. An early report showed that there is an association between cold-knife conisation and adverse obstetric outcomes, including preterm delivery [10]. The findings of a published meta-analysis have shown that pregnant women previously treated by LLETZ are at approximately twice the risk of a preterm birth (delivery prior to 37 weeks) than pregnant women in general. Additionally, they have a 1.7–3.7 fold risk of low birth weight and premature rupture of the membranes compared with untreated women [1, 11, 12]. The largest to date, a Norwegian study looking at preterm deliveries before and after LLETZ treatment, found the proportion of preterm deliveries in each group, respectively, to be 6.7% and 17.2% [13].

By contrast, there is limited data on the fertility and reproductive performance of women treated by LLETZ [14] with no strong association between cervical conisation or ablation and subfertility [13, 15].

Furthermore, studies have shown that excisional treatments for CIN or very early stage cancer (stage 1A) can lead to a small risk of complications in future pregnancies including [11, 15–17]:

- A higher risk of a baby that weighs less than 2.5 kg (low birthweight)
- An increase in Caesarean section delivery

As we know, connective tissue, smooth muscle, blood vessels and elastic fibres, which comprise the cervix, are considered to play an important role in pregnancy and delivery. Excessive tissue excision leads to a loose cervix or cervical incompetence, which could result in a higher rate of premature birth, miscarriage and increase the risk of infection.

Some bacteria associated with preterm birth, such as *Bacteroides fragilis* and Group B Streptococcus, can release phospholipase A2 or proteolytic enzymes, which are associated with uterine contractions and premature rupture of the membranes [16, 18].

There are many other risk factors for preterm delivery and premature birth in women who had excisional treatment for CIN. This could be due to a higher frequency of health problems when compared to the general population. Consequently, their increased risk of preterm delivery might be related to these factors [17]. One of the main risk factors is smoking, which plays a role in persistence of Human Papilloma Virus (HPV) infection through the impairment of the immune system [19]. Published literature has shown that women are more likely to experience a preterm delivery not only due to the loss of cervical tissue and the mechanical support that it provides [1, 10], but also because of the changes in the immune system and vaginal environment of women during pregnancy [14, 20]. These changes play a very important role in the persistence of HPV, which leads to the development of frequent ascending infections, increasing the risk of premature delivery.

3.1.2 Loop Depth and the Risk of Preterm Labour

There is agreement that the risk of premature birth increases with the depth of the excision [21]. The risk of preterm delivery (delivery < 37 weeks) was reported to increase by three fold when the depth of the loop increases from 10–12 mm to > 20 mm [14]. The risk is increased by both excisional and destructive procedures, but women who undergo excisional procedures are more likely to experience obstetric sequelae including a 6.1% risk of preterm rupture of membranes (PROM) in women who had LLETZ compared to the 3.4% risk of PROM in women who did not have LLETZ treatment [14, 21].

3.1.3 Cervical Length Screening

Serial cervical length measurement in mid-trimester is recommended in post-conisation/ post-LLETZ pregnancy to estimate the risk of spontaneous preterm birth [16, 21]. A short cervix of (<25 mm) is a strong predictor of preterm labour [16, 21].

Prophylactic cervical cerclage is recommended for pregnant women who have had a previous LLETZ or cone biopsy when the length of the cervix is less than 25 mm on a transvaginal ultrasound scan, which has been carried out between 16+0 and 24+0 weeks of pregnancy [22]. In non-pregnant treated women contemplating pregnancy, the role of prophylactic laparoscopic cervical cerclage with subsequent Caesarean delivery needs to be discussed.

3.2 Abnormal Smears

3.2.1 Introduction

The incidence of invasive cervical cancer in pregnancy is low with reported incidence rates ranging from 0.05% to 0.1% [23], and pregnancy itself does not have an adverse effect on the prognosis [23]. Furthermore, pregnancy is not a factor for worsening cervical lesions [24].

The cervical changes that occur during pregnancy can complicate the interpretation of cervical cytology and colposcopy [1, 23].

These changes include [1, 22]:

1 Increased blood supply with more pronounced vascular patterns
2 Increased production of mucous
3- Changes in the shape of the cervix – eversion of the cervix with lateral extension of the transformation zone

For these reasons, colposcopic evaluation requires a high degree of skill in pregnant women. It is at the clinicians discretion to decide if women who are seen in early pregnancy require a further assessment in the late second trimester [22, 23]. It is important that senior colposcopists with experience in interpreting colposcopic findings in pregnancy undertake the management of these women.

The National Health Service Cervical Screening Programme (NHSCSP) [22] has devised recommendations for cervical screening in pregnant women (Table 3.1).

3.2.2 Abnormal Smears and Colposcopy during Pregnancy

Pregnant women who meet the criteria for colposcopy should be examined in the colposcopy clinic, where the primary aim is to exclude invasive disease and to confirm the safety of deferring biopsy or treatment until the post-partum period [22].

Table 3.1 Cervical screening in pregnancy (NHSCSP)

- **If a woman has been called for routine screening and she is pregnant** – reschedule the test for when she is at least three months' post-partum
- **If a previous test was abnormal and in the interim the woman becomes pregnant** – colposcopy should not be delayed
  - Women may undergo colposcopy in late first or early second trimester, unless there is a clinical contraindication; however, for low-grade changes, the assessment may be delayed until after delivery
  - Women seen in early pregnancy may require a further assessment in the late second trimester

If a cervical biopsy is indicated during pregnancy, it does not usually affect the pregnancy. The absence of histological invasion cannot be guaranteed by a punch biopsy only and if a loop biopsy is performed. There is 25% risk of haemorrhage for biopsies taken during pregnancy by a diathermy loop [25], which is why it should be performed in a setting where there are facilities to manage haemorrhage and where a vaginal pack can be inserted post procedure. A general anaesthetic may be appropriate in some cases.

Studies have shown high rates of recurrence for both low-grade squamous intra-epithelial lesions and high-grade intra-epithelial lesions 2–5 years after diagnosis in the antepartum period [26, 27].

3.3 Cervical Cancer in Pregnancy

3.3.1 Introduction

Of women diagnosed with cervical cancer, 1–3% are pregnant women or post-partum, with half of these cases being diagnosed pre-natally and the other half being diagnosed in the 12 months after delivery [28].The rate of cervical cancer associated with pregnancy has declined in countries that conduct population-based cervical screening programmes like the United Kingdom and Sweden. Data from Sweden showed a reduction in cervical cancer during pregnancy from 1.4% to 0.9% following the application of a cervical screening programme [29]. Pregnant women with borderline nuclear changes or low-grade dyskaryosis rarely have high-grade changes at colposcopy that require biopsy during pregnancy [22–24].

There is currently no gold standard treatment for the management of invasive cervical cancer in pregnancy, which remains extremely challenging and requires a multi-disciplinary team discussion to optimise the treatment for the patient, in addition to simultaneously providing the best chance of survival for the baby [23].

The approach is based mainly on multiple factors including gestational age at the time of the diagnosis, stage of the disease, histological subtype, the future fertility desire and quality of life [23].

The symptoms of cervical cancer in pregnancy include painless vaginal bleeding, abnormal vaginal discharge, post coital bleeding and dyspareunia. If these symptoms occur, it is mandatory to undertake a speculum and pelvic examination and refer for colposcopy regardless of gestational age [29, 30].

Colposcopic features in invasive cancer do not differ from outside pregnancy with abnormal vessels, mosaic and punctuation along with irregular contours.

In patients with histological or colposcopic diagnosis of high-grade CIN (HGCIN), review in the colposcopy clinic should be undertaken at least every 12 weeks and if there is suspicion of disease progression then a repeat biopsy should be undertaken to exclude invasion. If highly suspicious of invasive cervical cancer, cervical cold-knife conisation or a LLETZ can be undertaken.

3.3.2 Staging of Cancer

MRI)= is the first line for staging of cervical cancer in pregnancy [31]. CT may be required where advanced disease such as lung or pleural spread is suspected but should only be undertaken where it is deemed the benefits will outweigh the risk to the fetus of ionising radiation.

3.3.3 Treatment

Treatment will depend on the stage of the cancer, gestational age and wishes of the patient:

IA – For early stage 1A1 cancers of the cervix, a LLETZ procedure will be sufficient and can be undertaken in pregnancy with all of the precautions stated previously to avoid haemorrhage. Consideration should be given to a prophylactic cervical cerclage procedure at the same time.

IA2/IB –For non-pregnant patients, a radical trachelectomy versus a radical hysterectomy is usually the preferred method of treatment depending on the patient's wishes to conserve fertility. However, in pregnancy, radical resection of the cervix is not recommended and consideration in this case will need to be given to a termination followed by treatment. If the patient does not wish a termination and depending on the gestational age, neoadjuvant chemotherapy (NACT) can be given.

This can also be used for higher stage tumours in order to treat and control the disease whilst fetal maturation is attained. The mainstay of NACT is carboplatin as a first-line chemotherapeutic agent [32]. It is not recommended beyond 34 weeks gestation and consideration should be given at this stage to administering steroids for fetal lung maturity and a Caesarean section or radical Caesarean hysterectomy [33].

Breastfeeding is contraindicated as the drugs can cross into breast milk and cause neonatal leucopenia [34].

The route of delivery is determined by the presence or absence of a visible tumour. If the tumour is still present, Caesarean delivery is preferred due to the risk of cancer cell implantation into the episiotomy scar [35].

3.4 Benign Cervical Lesions in Pregnancy

A common cause of painless vaginal bleeding, discharge or post-coital bleeding in pregnancy not associated with smear abnormalities is that due to cervical polyps. They are usually benign and may either be diagnosed as an incidental finding on a speculum examination or because they present with symptoms. In either case, the removal of either decidual or endocervical polyps seems associated with an increased risk of pregnancy loss and preterm birth and should ideally be managed conservatively during the pregnancy with the aim of removal post-partum if necessary [36].

Clinical Governance Issues

- It is important to keep in mind the possibility of cervical abnormalities in pregnant women who present with bleeding or abnormal discharge in pregnancy, and a clinical examination including a speculum examination and referral for colposcopy should be undertaken
- Thorough counselling regarding the risk of cervical incompetence and preterm labour should be undertaken prior to excisional treatment for pre-invasive disease and ablative methods should be considered if appropriate
- Consideration should be given to cervical cerclage in pregnant women where serial cervical length scans show shortening of the cervix
- Abnormal smears should warrant a colposcopy and possible biopsy to rule out invasive disease. Serial colposcopic examinations should be undertaken in every trimester by an

experienced colposcopist with the object being to manage high-grade, pre-invasive lesions conservatively until delivery and to detect invasive cancer
- In the case of cervical cancers detected in pregnancy, the management will be dictated by the gestation, stage of tumour and the patient's wishes as regards continuing the pregnancy. Any discussion needs to be undertaken with empathy
- Treatment with NACT should be considered in order to give time for fetal maturity

References

1 M. Kyrgiou, G. Koliopoulos, P. Martin-Hirsch, et al. Obstetric outcomes after conservative treatment for intraepithelial or early invasive cervical lesions: Systematic review and meta-analysis RID B-6887-2009. *Lancet,* **367** (2006), 489–98.

2 M. Quinn, P. Babb, J. Jones, et al. Effect of screening on incidence of and mortality from cancer of cervix in England: Evaluation based on routinely collected statistics. *BMJ,* **318** (1999), 904–8.

3 A. Moscicki, M. Schiffman, S. Kjaer and L. L. Villa. Updating the natural history of HPV and anogenital cancer. *Vaccine,* **24** (2006), 42–51.

4 T. C. Wright Jr, L. S. Massad and C. J. Dunton, et al. 2006 consensus guidelines for the management of women with cervical intraepithelial neoplasia or adenocarcinoma in situ. *Obstetrics & Gynecology,* **197** (2007), 340–5.

5 C. Chen, Y. Xu, W. Huang, Y. Du and C. Hu. Natural history of histologically confirmed high-grade cervical intraepithelial neoplasia during pregnancy: Meta-analysis. *BMJ Open,* **11** (2021), e048055.

6 L. Lancucki, ed. *Cervical Screening Programme, England: 2005–06.* (NHS Information Centre, 2006). https://bmjopen.bmj.com/content/11/8/e048055

7 W. Prendiville, J. Cullimore and S. Norman. Large loop excision of the transformation zone (LLETZ). A new method of management for women with cervical intraepithelial neoplasia. *British Journal of Obstetrics and Gynaecology,* **96** (1989), 1054–60.

8 T. C. Wright Jr, J. T. Cox, L. S. Massad, et al. 2001 consensus guidelines for the management of women with cervical intraepithelial neoplasia. *American Journal of Obstetrics and Gynecology,* **189** (2003), 295–304.

9 A. Herbert and J. A. Smith. Cervical intraepithelial neoplasia grade III (CIN III) and invasive cervical carcinoma: The yawning gap revisited and the treatment of risk. *Cytopathology,* **10** (1999), 161–70.

10 D. Andía, F. Mozo de Rosales, A. Villasante, et al. Pregnancy outcome in patients treated with cervical conization for cervical intraepithelial neoplasia. *International Journal of Gynecology & Obstetrics,* **112** (2011), 225–8.

11 M. Arbyn, M. Kyrgiou, C. Simoens, et al. Perinatal mortality and other severe adverse pregnancy outcomes associated with treatment of cervical intraepithelial neoplasia: Meta-analysis RID B-6887-2009. *BMJ,* **337** (2008), a1284.

12 F. Gkrozou, L. Antoun, R. Risk, et al. The risk of preterm delivery following large loop excision of the cervix: An observational cohort study. *Clinics in Surgery,* **5** (2021), 1–6.

13 M. Jakobsson, M. Gissler, A. Tiitinen, et al. Treatment for cervical intraepithelial neoplasia and subsequent IVF deliveries. *Human Reproduction,* **23** (2008), 2252–5.

14 M. Hein, A. C. Petersen, R. B. Helmig, et al. Immunoglobulin levels and phagocytes in the cervical mucus plug at term of pregnancy. *Acta Obstetrica et Gynecologia Scandinavica,* **84** (2005), 734–42.

15 C. L. Werner, J. Y. Lo, T. Heffernan, et al. Loop electrosurgical excision procedure

and risk of preterm birth. *Obstetrics & Gynecology,* **115** (2010), 605–8.

16 K. P. Himes and H. N. Simhan. Time from cervical conization to pregnancy and preterm birth. *Obstetrics & Gynecology,* **109** (2007), 314–319.

17 R. L. Fischer, G. Sveinbjornsson and C. Hansen. Cervical sonography in pregnant women with a prior cone biopsy or loop electrosurgical excision procedure. *Ultrasound in Obstetrics & Gynecology,* **36** (2010), 613–17.

18 C. Simoens, F. Goffin, P. Simon, et al. Adverse obstetrical outcomes after treatment of precancerous cervical lesions: A Belgian multicentre study. *British Journal of Obstetrics and Gynaecology,* **119** (2012), 1247–55.

19 A. Castanon, P. Brocklehurst, H. Evans, et al. Risk of preterm birth after treatment for cervical intraepithelial neoplasia among women attending colposcopy in England: Retrospective-prospective cohort study. *British Medical Journal,* **16** (2012), e5174.

20 W. T. Turlington, B. D. Wright and J. L. Powell. Impact of the loop electrosurgical excision procedure on future fertility. *Journal of Reproductive Medicine,* **41** (1996), 815–18.

21 M. Kyrgiou, A. Athanasiou, M. Paraskevaidi, et al. Adverse obstetric outcomes after local treatment for cervical preinvasive and early invasive disease according to cone depth: Systematic review and meta-analysis. *British Medical Journal,* **354** (2016), i3633.

22 National Institute for Health and Care Excellence. *Preterm Labour and Birth [Nice Guidelines NG25].* (2019). www.nice.org.uk/guidance/ng25

23 M. La Russa and A. R. Jeyarajah. Invasive cervical cancer in pregnancy. *Best Practice & Research Clinical Obstetrics & Gynaecology,* **33** (2016), 44–57, doi:10.1016/j.bpobgyn.2015.10.002. Epub 2015 Oct 23

24 D. K. Hong, S. A. Kim, K. T. Lim, et al. Clinical outcome of high-grade cervical intraepithelial neoplasia during pregnancy: A 10-year experience. *European Journal of Obstetrics & Gynecology and Reproductive Biology,* **236** (2019), 173–6. Epub 2019 Mar 25. PMID: 30933887. https://doi.org/10.1016/j.ejogrb.2019.03.023

25 N. Reed, J. Balega, T. Barwick, et al. British Gynaecological Cancer Society (BGCS) cervical cancer guidelines: Recommendations for practice. *European Journal of Obstetrics & Gynecology and Reproductive Biology,* **256** (2021), 433–65.

26 K. J. Kaplan, L. A. Dainty, B. Dolinsky, et al. Prognosis and recurrence risk for patients with cervical squamous intraepithelial lesions diagnosed during pregnancy. *Cancer,* **102** (2004), 228–32.

27 S. Ackermann, C. Gehrsitz, G. Mehlhorn, et al. Management and course of histologically verified cervical carcinoma in situ during pregnancy. *Acta Obstetrica et Gynecologica,* **85** (2006), 1134–7.

28 C. Nguyen, F. J. Montz and R. E. Bristow. Management of stage 1 cervical cancer in pregnancy. *Obstetrical & Gynecological Survey,* **55** (2000), 633–43.

29 B. Nitish, S. Zhujun, W. Dongchen, et al. Diagnosis and treatment of cervical cancer in pregnant women. *Cancer Medicine,* **8** (2019), 5425–30.

30 K. Van Calsteren, I. Vergote and F. Amant. *Cervical neoplasia during pregnancy: Diagnosis, management and prognosis. Best Practice & Research Clinical Obstetrics & Gynaecology,* **19** (2005), 611–30.

31 H. Hricak, C. B. Powell, K. K. Yu, et al. Invasive cervical carcinoma: Role of MR imaging in pretreatment work up costs minimisation and diagnostic efficacy analysis. *Radiology,* **198** (1996), 403–9.

32 K. N. Moore, T. J. Herzog, S. Lewin, et al. A comparison of cisplatin/paclitaxel and carboplatin/paclitaxel in stage IVB, recurrent or persistent cervical cancer. *Gynaecologic Oncology,* **105** (2007), 299–303.

33 A. Karam, N. Feldman, C. Holschneider, et al. Neoadjuvant cisplatin and

radical Caesarean hysterectomy for cervical cancer in pregnancy. *Nature Clinical Practice Oncology*, **4** (2007), 375–80.

34 P. C. Egan, M. E. Costanza, P. Dodlon, et al. Doxorubicin and cisplatin excretion into human milk. *Cancer Treatment Reports*, **69** (1985), 1387–9.

35 S. Alouni, K. Rida and P. Mathevet. Cervical cancer complicating pregnancy:

Implications of laparoscopic lymphadenectomy. *Gynecologic Oncology*, **108** (2008), 472–77.

36 G. Riemma, L. Della Corte, S. G. Vitale, et al. Surgical management of endocervical and decidual polyps during pregnancy: Systematic review and meta-analysis. *Archives of Gynecology and Obstetrics*, (2022), Epub. https://doi.org/10.1007/s00404-022-06550-z

Vulval Disorders in Pregnancy

David Nunns

4.1 Assessment of the Patient

4.1.1 History Taking

Most vulval skin diseases can be diagnosed on the basis of a history and clinical examination. An accurate description of symptoms and assessment of function are important to determine the impact of the condition on the patient. Table 4.1 outlines some key points to address in the history taking and the reasoning for them.

4.1.2 Vulval Examination

The normal vulva in an adult woman includes the mons pubis, inguinal folds, outer and inner labia (majora and minora), clitoris (body and hood), perineum, vestibule and anus (Figure 4.1). Hart's line is the junction between the vestibule and the inner labia and marks a change in epithelium type from mucosal type to stratified squamous. Vulval pathology may be a manifestation of a general skin condition and therefore, a complete skin examination to include the umbilicus, natal cleft, oral cavity, eyes and mouth should be performed if relevant. This allows a more complete assessment of disease extent and diagnosis especially for diseases that are not solely restricted to the vulval region such as psoriasis, eczema, lichen sclerosus and erosive lichen planus. It is important to note that the classical appearances of skin conditions may not apply to the vulval area as it is a covered, moist environment. Examination should be thorough and methodical to include all areas of the vulva, perineum and perianal area. The patient should initially be in the dorsal position for vulval and perineal examination and subsequently turned to the left lateral position to examine the perianal area. Good lighting is essential to view these areas adequately. It is not necessary for the patient to be placed in the lithotomy position.

Examination may show changes in the colour and texture of vulval skin or mucosa:

- *Erythema*' refers to reddening of the skin, which may be poorly demarcated, as in eczema or well demarcated, as in psoriasis. The presence of erythema usually indicates an underlying inflammatory process. If present in association with pain, infection should be considered
- *Whitening* of the skin may occur in the presence of a normal epidermis such as in vitiligo, or in conjunction with epidermal change such as lichen sclerosus
- *Lichenification* is the term used to describe a leathery thickening of the skin with increased skin markings which occurs in response to persistent rubbing. The vulval region is often moist and scaling is a less reliable sign than on other areas of the skin. It is most reliable on the mons pubis where scaling may be a manifestation of

Table 4.1 Vulval history taking points

Question	Reasoning
What are the key symptoms and how severe are they?	Itch can suggest skin disease or infection. Pain can be secondary to itching from skin damage through trauma. Vaginal discharge may suggest infection such as candidiasis
How long have the symptoms been present?	Acute symptoms may indicate infections such as vulvovaginal thrush or contact dermatitis. Chronic symptoms may be due to lichen sclerosus or lichen planus
What is the impact on the patient's function? ('How do the symptoms affect you?' or 'What do you miss as a result of the problem?')	Improvement in function (including sex) is an important clinical outcome
What treatments have been tried (including over the counter agents)?	The history should explore failed treatments, e.g. topical steroid frequency and amount as under usage with these treatments is common due to steroid phobia or a lack of understanding by the patient. Inappropriate topical treatments can exacerbate symptoms and potentially cause an irritant reaction
How is the patient cleaning the vulval area?	Over-washing may lead to skin damage and further irritation
Are there any possible contacts with irritants, e.g. soaps, shampoos, urine, and scented vaginal wipes?	These are potential irritants and can damage the skin potentially causing inflammation. Urine and scented vaginal wipes are potent skin irritants
Is there any systemic illness?	For example, diabetes, renal failure, anaemia (these may all be a cause of itch) or autoimmune conditions (higher chance of systemic autoimmunity in lichen sclerosus or erosive lichen planus)
Are there any other skin conditions present?	Skin disease at other skin sites may provide clues to the vulval diagnosis. For example, eczema or psoriasis. These may be very obvious, however signs may be subtle, for example psoriasis is sometimes hidden as cracking behind the ears, a scaly scalp or umbilical erythema

psoriasis. On other sites such as the natal cleft, scaling and lichenification may result in whiteness and splitting of the skin

The terms used to describe vulval lesions are described in Table 4.2.

4.1.3 Investigations

4.1.3.1 Diagnostic Vulval Biopsy

Outside of pregnancy, a 4mm Keyes punch biopsy is adequate and should ideally be carried out under local anaesthetic. A vulval biopsy is usually indicated for: 1) asymmetrical pigmented lesions, 2) persistently eroded areas, 3) indurated and suspicious

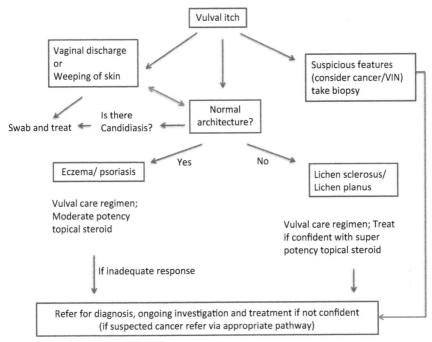

Fig 4.1 Algorithm for the management of vulval itching (c/o Dr Karen Gibbon)

ulcerated areas, 4) when there is poor response to treatment following the initial diagnosis. The site selected for biopsy should be tissue-representative of the lesion or area of abnormality. This is usually at the edge of the lesion and should also include some normal tissue. The most central area may be inflamed which may give minimal tissue diagnosis because of the inflammation present. In pregnancy there are understandable concerns that patients have with regards to biopsy. There is no evidence that a biopsy would compromise the pregnancy outcome.

4.1.3.2 Vaginal and Vulval Swabs

Infection with candidiasis is common in pregnancy and a swab should be considered. In patients with a pre-existing skin issue there should be a low threshold for taking a swab when there is a loss of symptom control in inflammatory dermatoses. This may be a reason why lichen sclerosus appears initially well controlled with potent steroids and then flares up. Minor degrees of skin trauma from scratching can produce infection. Occasionally, genital herpes can be a cause of vulval symptoms and a viral culture swab may be necessary.

4.1.3.3 The Vulval Clinic

As many vulval problems are chronic, rare and difficult, a multidisciplinary input may be required. Service provision can vary but most hospitals in the UK provide a local vulval clinic providing expert help. Members of the vulval service may include dermatology, genito-urinary medicine, physiotherapy, pain management, psychosexual therapy, pathology and urogynaecology.

Table 4.2 Terminology for lesions that may be seen in the vulval area

Lesion terminology	Description	Example
Fissure	A thin 'hairline' crack in the skin surface due to excessive dryness	Psoriasis and lichen sclerosus
Excoriation	Scratch mark, may be single or multiple	May be seen in any itchy skin condition, e.g. atopic eczema, lichen sclerosus
Erosion	A shallow denuded area due to loss of the epidermis (surface layer of skin)	Erosive lichen planus
Ulcer	Full thickness loss of the epidermis (top layer of skin) +/− dermis	Aphthous ulceration
Macule	Flat area of colour change	Vulval melanosis Ecchymosis (subcutaneous purpura) seen in lichen sclerosus
Nodule	Large palpable lesion greater than 0.5 cm in diameter	Squamous cell carcinoma, Scabies
Papule	Small palpable lesion less than 0.5 cm in diameter	Genital warts Molluscum contagiosum Seborrhoeic keratosis
Plaque	A palpable flat lesion greater than 0.5 cm diameter. It may be elevated or may be a thickened area without being visibly raised above the skin surface	Vulval intra-epithelial neoplasia Squamous cell carcinoma Large seborrheic keratosis
Vesicle	Small fluid filled blister less than 0.5 cm diameter	Bullous pemphigoid
Lichenification	An accentuation of skin markings commonly associated with thickening of epidermis usually caused by scratching or rubbing	Lichen simplex

4.1.4 Specific Vulval Skin Diseases

It is important to understand that vulval itch (sometimes termed 'pruritus vulvae') is a common presenting complaint. It is not in itself a diagnosis, but a symptom indicating an underlying cause. Itch may be the presenting symptom of many vulval skin disorders. It may also be related to an underlying systemic illness as part of a more generalised complaint of itch. Common dermatoses in the anogenital area can affect any female and include dermatitis (irritant, allergic contact or atopic), psoriasis and lichen sclerosis. Other local causes of anogenital itch include infections (candidiasis, viral warts), urinary or faecal incontinence, lichen simplex chronicus, squamous cell carcinoma and oestrogen deficiency. The algorithm outlined in Figure 4.1 is useful when assessing patients who present with vulval itch (courtesy of Dr Karen Gibbon).

Table 4.2 provides a summary of the clinical features of specific skin diseases, diagnosis and treatment and gives a framework for making a diagnosis, initial treatment and ongoing referral teams. With some conditions, for example, psoriasis, dermatologists will need to take a lead clinician role in management. We have included the important value of a general practitioner in management as they are usually responsible for the ongoing management of patients in the community.

4.2 Management of Vulval Skin Conditions

4.2.1 General Principles

The initial principles of management are the same for all vulval skin conditions and a holistic approach is required. Good education, support and counselling are needed with extra time given to addressing the disease process, discussing general vulval care measures and managing expectations. It is useful to provide information leaflets, direct patients to relevant patient-oriented websites and write down instructions for applying topical agents (see 'Additional resources' for sources of patient information). The use of a mirror or model in the clinic setting is helpful to show patients where to apply their topical treatments.

4.2.2 Correct Barrier Function

Most vulval skin conditions are characterised by skin or mucosal barrier breakdown as well as underlying inflammation. Correction of the epidermal barrier is important in helping to reduce inflammation. For washing, soap and other routine cleaning agents (e.g. wipes) should be avoided, as they are likely to act as irritants or allergens. Irritation from urinary and faecal incontinence needs to be addressed as these are a common cause of irritation and make underlying skin pathology worse. 'Soap substitution' with a bland cream or ointment-based emollient is best for cleansing. The same agent can then be used as a moisturiser to both provide a barrier to the site and sooth inflamed skin. There is no preferred emollient to use and the best one is the one the patient will adhere to. Emollient creams (not ointments) can be placed in the fridge as this can help sooth the skin.

4.2.3 Using Topical Steroids on the Vulva

Topical steroids reduce inflammation associated with skin diseases such as lichen planus, lichen sclerosus and eczema leading to improvement in symptoms and appearance. However, there are patient and physician concerns regarding the use of topical steroids due to issues surrounding side effects, particularly skin or mucosal atrophy, which can lead to undertreatment and less control of symptoms. It is important therefore to use the correct strength of topical steroid for the necessary length of time on the appropriate body site with clear instructions to the patient so that they can be confident in self-management and be reassured that when applied correctly 'skin thinning' is very unlikely. Mucosal surfaces such as the vulval vestibule are remarkably resistant to steroid atrophy.

4.3 Lichen Sclerosus

Lichen sclerosus is an autoimmune, chronic, inflammatory skin condition. On examination there may be porcelain white papules and plaques, ecchymoses (subcutaneous purpura), erosions (loss of epidermis), fissures and lichenification. There can be a 'figure of eight' appearance to the disease. Loss of normal anatomy, labial fusion and adhesions are late signs of disease. The diagnosis is made clinically if confident or using a vulval biopsy. Consider biopsy(s) if there are indurated or suspicious areas. The primary treatment includes superpotent topical steroids and emollients (see topical steroids and their use in the treatment of vulval skin conditions). These can be used in pregnancy. There is a small risk of cancer (less than 5% risk) so patients should be encouraged to self exam on a regular (suggested monthly) basis. A Cochrane systematic review showed there is reasonable randomised controlled trial evidence for the use of topical steroids in lichen sclerosus and The British Association of Dermatologists suggest the use of the superpotent topical steroid, clobetasol proprionate 0.05%, over a three-month reducing course (suggested daily for one month, alternate days for one month and twice a week maintenance) [1, 2]. In general, topical steroids should be used once-daily. There is no evidence to suggest that twice-daily application is superior, although twice-daily has greater potential to cause side effects. Ointments are preferable to creams as they contain fewer constituents and therefore have a lower chance of causing irritation/contact allergy. Once control of inflammation and symptoms has been achieved, topical steroids should be reduced to the minimum frequency required to maintain remission. Maintenance therapy is of value and with this schedule 30–60 g of topical steroid will be used on average per year. Topical steroids should only be used on affected areas to prevent side effects in adjacent skin. There are few studies to show the impact of the condition on disease control in pregnancy, but a normal vaginal delivery should be possible for the majority of patients. *There is no contraindication to using topical corticosteroids for symptomatic lichen sclerosus during pregnancy. One study reported topical corticosteroids requirements in pregnancy were the same pre-pregnancy and that as compliance with treatment fell postnatally patients became increasing symptomatic* [3].

4.4 Contact Dermatitis

Two types can affect the vulva: the *irritant form* (triggered by irritants, e.g. soap, urine) with poorly defined erythema present where the irritant has been applied; the *allergic form* where erythema extends outside of the area where the allergen has been applied and diagnosis is made based on clinical history and examination. Patch testing is used if allergic contact dermatitis suspected. Treatment is based on moderate (e.g. clobetasone butyrate 0.05%) or potent (e.g. mometasone furoate 0.1%) topical steroids plus emollients to gain control of the inflammation [4].

4.5 Candidiasis

Patients with vulvovaginal candidiasis typically complain of itching, burning or soreness on the vulva and characteristic features include dryness, erythema and swelling of the vulval skin. Superficial fissuring and ulceration, due to scratching, may also be seen. A curd-like white vaginal discharge may be present and this will be seen on examination with a Cusco's speculum. Culture of a high vaginal swab will usually confirm the presence of a yeast organism, the most common of which is *Candida albicans,* a normal commensal of the gut and vagina. *Candida glabrata* or *Candida tropicalis* are found in a small proportion of patients, and these organisms may be resistant to the commonly-used antifungals. A course of broad-spectrum antibiotics may lead to an acute episode of vulvovaginal candidiasis, which is also associated with sexual activity, pregnancy and the combined oral contraceptive pill.

Partners and asymptomatic patients do not require treatment. Antifungal therapy is with oral fluconazole (not in pregnancy) or with clotrimazole (topical cream and vaginal pessaries). A seven-day course of treatment is usually recommended, but longer courses may be required in pregnancy. Where a history of recurrent episodes is given (four or more per year), predisposing conditions such as diabetes should be ruled out. For patients taking the combined oral contraceptive pill, stopping this may be helpful, but ensure that an alternative form of contraception is in place before this takes place. For repeated infections, a prophylactic course of fluconazole 150 mg once weekly for six months may be considered [5].

4.6 Bartholin Gland Cysts

There are two Bartholin glands situated within the labia majora on both sides, with their ducts opening into the vestibule at the 4 and 8 o'clock positions. They have the function of producing mucous for lubrication during intercourse. They are unusual in that they have a long duct from the main body of the gland, which may become blocked to produce a deep-seated cystic swelling in the region of the gland that histologically is lined by mucinous epithelium. A Bartholin gland cyst is diagnosed clinically. Small cysts are often asymptomatic and can be managed conservatively. Some patients may complain of the feeling of a lump or pain during intercourse. Traditionally, symptomatic cysts are managed surgically with marsupialisation during which the cyst wall is incised and the edge sutured so there is a continuous surface from the interior to the exterior enabling the interior to drain. This procedure has a high cure rate. Another option involving insertion of a Word catheter into the cyst has been advocated and can be carried out in the outpatient setting [6]: Under local anaesthesia, a small balloon with an inflatable distal end is inserted into the cyst cavity. The aim of the balloon catheter insertion is to create an epithelialised fistula or sinus tract to allow drainage. The catheter has a stem (3 cm long) and an inflatable balloon tip to hold saline, which allows the catheter to remain in the cyst cavity. There is no good clinical evidence to support either technique. In pregnancy, there is a place for conservative management and patient reassurance with a post-natal review.

Cysts may become infected with *Escherichia coli*, creating a Bartholin gland abscess. The management of a Bartholin gland abscess involves incision and drainage of the abscess, usually with an incision on the inner side of the vestibule, even in pregnancy. If an abscess spontaneously discharges, then there is less value in incision and drainage and the abscess should slowly resolve. Routine antibiotics are not usually necessary.

4.7 Vulvodynia

Vulvodynia has been defined by the International Society for the Study of Vulval Diseases (ISSVD) as vulval discomfort, most often described as a burning pain, occurring in the absence of relevant visible findings or a specific, clinically identifiable neurologic disorder [7].

The ISSVD classifies vulvodynia according to site (generalised or localised), requirement of stimulus (provoked, unprovoked or mixed) and onset (primary or secondary). Patients with provoked pain were formerly diagnosed as having 'vestibulitis', which is incorrect as there is no inflammatory component to the condition. The most common types of vulvodynia are localised provoked vulval pain (vestibulodynia) and generalised unprovoked vulval pain. It is worth mentioning that in clinical practice some patients will have a combination of both unprovoked and provoked pain, which is not reflected in the literature.

Vulvodynia is a diagnosis of exclusion and a thorough history and examination are essential to confidently exclude subtle skin disease. A pain history should include nature, severity, site, aggravating or relieving factors. One important differential is pudendal neuralgia, which is a nerve entrapment syndrome of the pudendal nerve. These patients usually experience pain on sitting, relieved by lying down or standing. They may also complain of the sensation of a 'lump or egg' being present in the vagina. An assessment of the impact of pain on function is important and a psychosexual history should be explored if appropriate. For women with provoked pain, dyspareunia is a main complaint and can often be missed in the initial referral. Vulvodynia can lead to secondary psychosexual problems such as avoidance, phobia of touch, loss of libido and vaginismus. Recognition of this as the main problem for the patient is crucial so that treatment can focus on sexual rehabilitation either through self-management (increasing communication with partners, use of lubricants and vaginal dilators) or more formal treatment with a psychosexual counsellor.

The heterogeneity of vulvodynia poses a significant challenge to identifying any kind of 'gold standard' treatment and patients require individualised, combination treatment strategies. As with many chronic pain conditions, good quality evidence for management is limited [8]. It is important that a 'one size fits all' approach is avoided. Not every treatment will be suitable for every woman and certain interventions may be more suited to a particular type of vulvodynia, for example, topical lidocaine for localised provoked pain (vestibulodynia).

The optimal mode of delivery for women with vulvodynia is not defined and there is no strong evidence that the type of delivery will influence the development of recurrence of vulvodynia. There are likely to be concerns from patients who have provoked pain especially those who have had surgery.

4.8 Conclusions

An accurate diagnosis for women with vulval disease relies on a thorough history and detailed examination. The use of topical steroids in pregnancy is safe and patients are likely to require additional support and reassurance with use. Referral to a colleague with an interest in vulval disease is of value where there is doubt regarding the diagnosis, a biopsy indication or where treatment has been unsuccessful. The prognosis for women with vulval symptoms is good, providing that an accurate diagnosis has been made.

Further Resources

Dermnetnz: The Dermatology Resource www.dermnetnz.org
British Society for the Study of Vulval Disease www.bssvd.org
Online resource endorsed by the ISSVD http://vulvovaginaldisorders.com/
Online training course which is free to UK doctors to access www.e-lfh.org.uk/projects/dermatology/index.html

Clinical Governance Issues

- Women with vulval lichen sclerosus and vulval intra-epithelial neoplasia (VIN) have an approximately 3–5% lifetime risk of vulval cancer. It is important to tell patients to report the presence of any skin changes over time
- Documentation of lesions with a clear picture is helpful
- Description of lesions using dermatological descriptors, for example, macule, ulcers should be encouraged to encourage greater consistency of reporting
- If there is a suspicion of a vulval cancer please refer to the relevant gynaecologist. An outpatient biopsy is not contraindicated in pregnancy

References

1   S. M. Neill, F. M. Lewis, F. M. Tatnall and N. H. Cox. British Association of Dermatologists' guidelines for the management of lichen sclerosus 2010. *The British Journal of Dermatology,* **163** (2010), 672–82.

2   C. C. Chi, G. Kirtschig, M. Baldo, et al. Topical interventions for genital lichen sclerosus. *Cochrane Database of Systematic Reviews,* 7 (2011), CD008240. https://doi.org/10.1002/14651858.CD008240.pub2

3   Y. Nguyen, J. Bradford and G. Fischer. Lichen sclerosus in pregnancy: A review of 33 cases. *Australian & New Zealand Journal of Obstetrics & Gynaecology,* **58** (2018), 686–9.

4   S. M. O'Gorman and R. R. Torgerson. Allergic contact dermatitis of the vulva. *Dermatitis,* **24** (2013), 64–72.

5   National Institute for Health and Care Excellence. *Guidance on the Management of Vulvovaginal Candidiasis.* https://cks.nice.org.uk/topics/candida-female-genital/

6   Z. Haider, G. Condous, E. Kirk, et al. The simple outpatient management of Bartholin's abscess using the Word catheter: A preliminary study. *Australian & New Zealand Journal of Obstetrics & Gynaecology,* **47** (2007), 137–40.

7   J. Bornstein, A. T. Goldstein, C. K. Stockdale, et al. Consensus vulvar pain terminology committee of the International Society for the Study of Vulvovaginal Disease (ISSVD), the International Society for the Study of Women's Sexual Health (ISSWSH), and the International Pelvic Pain Society (IPPS). *Journal of Lower Genital Tract Disease,* **20** (2016), 126–30.

8   D. Nunns, D. Mandal, M. Byrne, et al. British Society for the Study of Vulval Disease (BSSVD) Guideline Group. Guidelines for the management of vulvodynia. *British Journal of Dermatology,* **162** (2010), 1180–5.

Congenital Uterine Malformations and Vaginal Anomalies

Bibi Zeyah Fatemah Sairally, Pallavi Latthe

5.1 Introduction

Congenital uterine malformations of the female genital tract are deviations from normal anatomy due to the embryological maldevelopment of one or both Müllerian ducts [1]. They are often asymptomatic with an estimated prevalence of 5.5% [2] in the general population and encompass a wide range of anomalies such as uterine agenesis, unicornuate uterus, bicornuate uterus, didelphys uterus or septate uterus, amongst others. Most are asymptomatic unless they present with amenorrhoea and pain but they have also been linked with some negative pregnancy outcomes such as recurrent miscarriages, infertility, preterm labour or malpresentation.

5.1.1 Classification of Congenital Female Genital Tract Malformations

There have been several systems proposed for the classification of female genital tract anomalies. In recent years, the most commonly used system proposed by the American Society of Reproductive Medicine (ASRM), where the anomalies are sorted using an embryological-clinical classification [3], has been superseded by the joint consensus between the European Society of Human Reproduction and Embryology (ESHRE) and the European Society for Gynaecological Endoscopy (ESGE), which was developed through a structured Delphi process [4].

The ESHRE/ESGE [4] classification system describes female genital anomalies anatomically (uterine, cervix and vagina) as well as grading them embryologically and provides a seven-category classification system (U0–U6) for congenital uterine anomalies (CUAs) as shown in Figure 5.1.

Class U0 is a normal uterus while U1 describes a dysmorphic uterus with a normal uterine outline but with an abnormal shape of the uterine cavity excluding any septa. Class U2 incorporates a septate uterus where the Müllerian ducts have merged but there is an incomplete resorption of the middle septum. The latter is defined as a normal uterine outline with an internal indentation of more than 50% of the uterine wall thickness. U3 or bicorporeal uterus is due to the incomplete fusion of the Müllerian ducts giving an abnormal uterine outline with an external indentation of more than 50% of the uterine wall thickness. Class U4 describes a hemi-uterus where there is a unilaterally formed functional uterus with either a rudimentary horn or an absent contralateral aspect. U5 or aplastic uterus is uterine aplasia with the complete absence of a cavity or the presence of a rudimentary horn. Class U6 is reserved for all unclassified cases that do not fit the other groups [4].

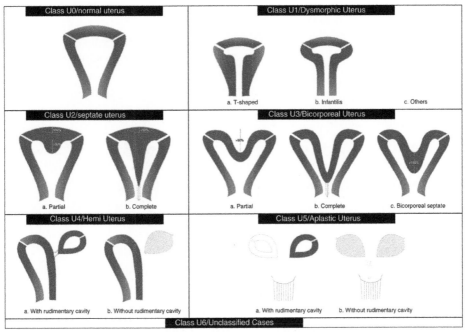

Fig 5.1 ESHRE/ESGE classification of uterine anomalies (reproduced with permission from Grimbizis et al. [4])

The diagnosis of CUAs has evolved with 3D transvaginal scanning (TVS) and MRI imaging showing superiority over previous conventional imaging such as 2D TVS, hysterosalpingography (HSG) and sonohysterography [5–8]. Indeed, the previous gold standard of combined hysteroscopy and laparoscopy has now been replaced by 3D ultrasound (preferably transvaginal) and a gynaecological examination, which is less invasive and can still classify the different uterine phenotypes correctly [4, 8].

In this chapter, we will be looking at a range of congenital female genital tract anomalies and their individual effect on pregnancy as well as specific considerations for each in the antenatal, intrapartum and post-natal periods. This will include septate uterus, bicornuate uterus, didelphys uterus and vaginal septum. We will also explore the same issues for previous repair or surgery of the congenital anomalies and will explore the approach to counselling women with these complications.

5.2 Septate Uterus

The ESHRE/ESGE defines the septate uterus as a uterus with a normal outline but with an internal indentation at the midline exceeding 50% of the uterine wall thickness [4]. It is a canalisation defect which can also sometimes extend through the whole uterus into the cervix and vagina. An arcuate/normal uterus, even though absent from the ESHRE/ESGE classification, was described by the ASRM in 2016 as an indentation depth from interstitial to apex of less than 1 cm with an indentation angle of more than 90 degrees, while a septate uterus was defined as an indentation depth from interstitial to apex of more than 1.5 cm with an indentation angle of less than 90 degrees [9]. Criticisms of

Table 5.1 Complications and associated risk ratios for subseptate, septate and arcuate uteri (from Chan et al. and Venetis et al., with permission) [13, 14]

Complications	Risk ratio (95% confidence interval) *Statistically significant
Subseptate or septate uterus	
Clinical pregnancy rate	0.86 (0.77–0.96) *
First trimester miscarriage	2.89 (2.02–4.14) *
Second trimester miscarriage	2.22 (0.74–6.65)
Preterm birth rate	2.14 (1.48–3.11) *
Fetal malpresentation at delivery	6.24 (4.05–9.62) *
Fetal growth restriction	2.54 (1.04–6.23) *
Arcuate uterus	
Second trimester miscarriage	2.39 (1.33–4.27) *
Fetal malpresentation at delivery	2.53 (1.54–4.18) *

overdiagnosis of a septate uterus have been reported with the ESHRE/ESGE classification compared to the ASRM criteria as there is a lack of evidence to support improved reproductive outcomes for those originally identified as having a normal uterus compared to those reclassified as having a septate uterus when using the ESHRE/ESGE classification [10, 11]. Most of the evidence available on septate and arcuate uterus are based on the definition used by the ASRM which will therefore be the one employed in this chapter.

Having a septate uterus has been associated with the worst reproductive outcome of all the other uterine anomalies with a term live birth rate of 30% [12]. A systematic review by Chan et al. has shown that women with canalisation defects such as septate and a subseptate uteri have a reduction in clinical pregnancy rate, increase in first trimester miscarriage, significant increase in preterm birth rate as well as an increased rate of fetal malpresentation at delivery [13]. Interestingly, the same systematic review also identified having an arcuate uterus as an increased risk for having a second trimester miscarriage compared to having a normal uterus, while a septate uterus showed no effect on second trimester miscarriage rates. Women with an arcuate uterus also had an increased rate of fetal malpresentation at delivery [13]. A meta-analysis by Venetis et al. also identified a statistically significant association between a septate uterus and the possibility of fetal growth restriction [14]. These complications and associated risk ratios are stated in Table 5.1.

The surgical intervention of choice for a septate uterus is hysteroscopic metroplasty or hysteroscopic transcervical resection of the uterine septum. A randomised controlled trial (RCT) comparing hysteroscopic septum resection with conservative management in women with a septate uterus has not as yet been completed [15]. However, the National Institute for Health and Care Excellence (NICE) has advised offering hysteroscopic metroplasty to women with a septate uterus who have suffered adverse reproductive outcomes such as recurrent miscarriage or primary infertility [16, 17].

Management plan for septate uterus:

- Pre-pregnancy counselling could be considered for women who have a known CUA
- Consultant-led care throughout pregnancy
- Serial ultrasound growth scans during the antenatal period
- Follow-up according to the national preterm birth care pathway
- Women with a first diagnosis of a CUA during the antenatal period will require follow-up renal tract scanning to rule out congenital renal anomalies which can be commonly associated with a CUA [18]
- While a normal vaginal delivery can be considered as the mode of delivery of choice, women should be made aware that there is a statistically significant increase in the overall Caesarean section delivery rate in women with minor fusion abnormality (arcuate, septate and T-shaped uteri) (p = 0.012), which may partially be explained by the increased risk of fetal malpresentation [19]
- Patients who have undergone a hysteroscopic transcervical resection of a uterine septum have no contraindication to undergoing a vaginal birth as long as the uterine cavity was not breached
- Women with known septate or arcuate uteri who have had a successful pregnancy and parturition do not require any specific post-partum follow-up. Women who have experienced any adverse reproductive outcomes should however be referred to a gynaecologist in the post-partum period for consideration of septum resection

5.3 Bicornuate, Didelphys and Unicornuate Uteri

Various degrees of unification defects of the paired Müllerian ducts result in either a bicornuate uterus, didelphys uterus or a unicornuate uterus. A bicorporeal uterus is defined as an external indentation at the fundal midline of more than 50% of the uterine wall thickness [4]. Additionally, a bicornuate or partial bicorporeal uterus is characterised by a division of the uterine corpus above the level of the cervix, whereas a didelphys or complete bicorporeal uterus is characterised by a division of the uterine corpus up to the level of the cervix [4]. A unicornuate uterus or hemi-uterus describes a unilateral uterine development with a rudimentary or absent contralateral part [4].

The systematic review by Chan at al. did not identify unification defects as having a clinically significant difference in pregnancy rates compared to women with a normal uterus but there was a significant association with preterm birth and a consistent significant increase in fetal malpresentation at birth [13].

In certain cases, increased risk of adverse pregnancy outcomes was identified depending on the unification defect in question. There was an increased risk of first trimester miscarriages in women with bicornuate and unicornuate uteri compared to a normal uterus [13]. Having a bicornuate uterus also doubled the risk of having a second trimester miscarriage compared to having a normal uterus [13]. In the study conducted by Venetis et al., women with didelphys, bicornuate and unicornuate uteri had a significantly higher probability of having a neonate of low birth weight (less than 2500 g) than women without a CUA [14]. A statistically significant association between a bicornuate uterus or didelphys uterus and the probability of fetal growth restriction was also identified [14]. The listed complications and associated risk ratios are shown in Table 5.2.

Table 5.2 Complications and associated risk ratios for different unification defects (from Chan et al. and Venetis et al., with permission) [13, 14]

Complications	Risk ratio (95% Confidence interval) * statistically significant
Unification defects (unicornuate, bicornuate and didelphys)	
Clinical pregnancy rate	0.87 (0.68–1.11)
Preterm birth rate	2.97 (2.08–4.23) *
Fetal malpresentation at delivery	3.87 (2.42–6.18) *
Bicornuate uterus	
First trimester miscarriage	3.40 (1.18–9.76) *
Second trimester miscarriage	2.32 (1.05–5.15) *
Low birth weight	1.74 (1.13–2.69) *
Fetal growth restriction	2.80 (1.06–7.34) *
Didelphys uterus	
Low birth weight	2.40 (1.40–4.11) *
Fetal growth restriction	4.94 (2.20–11.09) *
Unicornuate uterus	
First trimester miscarriage	2.15 (1.03–4.47) *
Low birth weight	3.54 (2.22–5.64) *

A retrospective cohort study by Fox et al. reported a significantly increased risk of pre-eclampsia in patients with unification defects (p = 0.014) [19]. The aetiology of this is not well-understood but it is known that CUAs may be associated with congenital renal anomalies (with unilateral renal agenesis being the commonest presentation) due to their similar embryological origin which may predispose them to having pre-eclampsia. There have also been some reported cases of second trimester uterine rupture in the literature in women presenting with a pregnancy in the rudimentary horn of a unicornuate uterus. Of note, a case series by Nahum et al. looked at 588 cases where 50% of patients presented with a uterine rupture even though no causal link was found for this [20].

Rarely, some women with bicornuate uterus or uterus didelphys undergo abdominal metroplasty. There is no significant improvement in obstetric outcomes even though the available data are scant and the procedure itself has a high rate of complications [1, 21]. However, this is not generally advised unless there is a significant adverse reproductive history that has already been investigated for a correctable endocrine or metabolic cause of pregnancy loss [21].

Management plan for unification defects:

- Consultant-led care and counselling with regards to the risks
- Follow-up antenatally by the UK Preterm Clinical Network so as to identify any signs of preterm birth early and offer the appropriate timely intervention such as a cervical cerclage

- Women identified with unification defects should have all the appropriate renal baseline investigations during the antenatal period or pre-pregnancy. This should include a kidney function test and urinary tract ultrasound scan as a minimum
- Serial ultrasound growth scans during the antenatal period for bicornuate and didelphys uteri
- High index of clinical suspicion if a woman with a CUA presents acutely to maternity triage or the emergency department with abdominal pain and free fluid to rule out pregnancy in a rudimentary horn
- Women identified as having small-for-gestational-age babies (SGA) or fetal growth restricted (FGR) babies should be continually monitored throughout labour
- A vaginal delivery can be aimed for but women should be made aware of the increased risk of fetal malpresentation and potential need for Caesarean section
- If an abdominal metroplasty has been performed, a Caesarean section delivery is indicated due to the high risk of uterine rupture
- The post-partum period is usually no different to that of the general population

5.4 Vaginal Septum and Repair

Vaginal anomalies include longitudinal and transverse vaginal septae and may be obstructing or non-obstructing in nature [4]. The longitudinal vaginal septum is formed by incomplete resorption of the fused Müllerian ducts, while the transverse vaginal septum occurs due to the failure of canalisation of the vaginal plate or due to a lack of vertical fusion of the Müllerian duct with the urogenital sinus [22]. Longitudinal non-obstructing vaginal septum is usually a variant of a septate or bicorporeal uterus with a septate or double cervices, while a longitudinal obstructing vaginal septum may cause the presence of an obstructing hemi-vagina but similarly presenting with uterus didelphys or a septate uterus along with an ipsilateral renal anomaly or agenesis [22]. Transverse septae can be perforate or imperforate as well as vary in their thickness and location in the vagina [23]. Unlike uterine anomalies, most vaginal anomalies tend to be diagnosed and treated prior to procreation and hence, most of the reproductive outcome data available are following surgical intervention. Early diagnosis and surgical intervention for vaginal anomalies help to reduce long-term morbidity but this relies on the accurate diagnosis through clinical examination, ultrasound scanning and the use of MRI [24].

Longitudinal obstructing vaginal septae have a conception rate of 55% [25]. Rock et al. showed that women undergoing vaginal excision for obstructing longitudinal vaginal septum did not have a fertility concern with six out of seven women they observed successful in conceiving [26]. Similarly, Haddad et al. conducted a reproductive question-naire 6.5 years following vaginal septum excision showing that nine out of nine people attempting a pregnancy were successful with a total of 20 pregnancies achieved [27].

Williams et al. reported a 100% (7 total) pregnancy success rate following the vaginal excision of a thin transverse vaginal septum, out of which one took more than one year to conceive [23]. On the other hand, Rock et al. reported a significantly reduced chance of conception following resection of a transverse vaginal septum compared to an imperforate hymen (47% versus 86%, $p < 0.05$) with a low septae (4 out of 4) showing better pregnancy outcomes than a mid (3 out of 7) or a high septae (2 out of 8) [28]. The cause is still uncertain but is thought to be due to a combination of the rate of stenosis and endometriosis depending on the location of the transverse septae, the surgical approach employed and the timing of diagnosis and subsequent intervention [28, 29]. In those women that do manage to conceive and carry the pregnancy, the most common obstetric complications encountered seem to be vaginal soft tissue dystocia increasing the risk of an emergency Caesarean section or lateral vault lacerations [29].

Joki-Erkkila et al. looked at the long-term sequalae of obstructing vaginal anomalies and compared the fertility and obstetric outcomes between imperforate hymen and longitudinal vaginal septae [22]. The successful birth rate following surgical intervention was 82% in the longitudinal group versus 94% in the transverse group [22]. Of note, there was a statistically significant lower birth weight in the longitudinal obstructing group compared to the transverse septae, likely due to the associated uterine abnormalities present in the longitudinal group [22]. There was also a higher Caesarean section rate noted in the longitudinal group (70% versus 60%) [22]; the reason for which was uncertain.

Management plan:

- In women with previous vaginal septum and repair, consultant-led care throughout the pregnancy would be advisable
- Serial growth scanning should be considered in women with previous longitudinal vaginal anomalies due to the high association of uterine abnormalities
- There should be a discussion with the woman about the risks of vaginal delivery including the small possibility of vaginal soft tissue dystocia with previous transverse septum repair and risks of vaginal lacerations
- A low level of clinical suspicion should be maintained if there is a delay in the first or second stage of labour so that senior input is obtained early

5.5 Counselling and Reproductive Outcomes

The majority of women with a CUA have a normal reproductive outcome. However, for the small proportion of women who do have adverse pregnancy implications, counselling and psychosocial support is of value alongside investigations and management options.

The increased risks in pregnancy are dependent on the type and severity of the CUAs but as previously discussed, those include first and second trimester miscarriages, preterm labour, fetal malpresentation, fetal growth restriction or low birth weight and pre-eclampsia. Those women might require serial fetal growth surveillance during the antenatal period as well as a follow-up for preterm birth screening and cervical cerclage.

The place of surgery is dependent on the type of anomaly that the patient presents with as well as their individual risk of adverse pregnancy outcome. Preoperatively, women should be informed of the evidence on the efficacy of the procedure planned as well as any risks associated with surgery.

The evidence supports hysteroscopic resection of a uterine septum in cases of recurrent miscarriages as well as infertility. Counselling is key prior to surgery so that patients are aware they may require more than one intervention and they may still experience adverse outcomes despite the adequacy of the uterine septum resection [30]. There is insufficient evidence to advocate a specific length of waiting time following surgery before attempting to conceive even though some observational studies suggest healing is completed after two months [31, 32].

Antenatally, any woman who has had previous surgical treatment would require consultant-led care during the subsequent pregnancy. The management of the patient would be dependent on their individual risk factors and may necessitate a multidisciplinary approach.

5.6 Conclusion

The current evidence available suggests that CUAs and vaginal anomalies, although uncommon, can have a significant impact on the reproductive outcome of a woman. It is therefore important to be aware of the steps that need to be taken to mitigate the risks.

All women with a diagnosed CUA will need consultant-led care and ideally should have an early antenatal consultation to discuss the associated risks and management plan prenatally and for the pregnancy. Obstetricians need to be aware of the different types of CUAs and vaginal anomalies, what to counsel women about in terms of risks as well as how to look after those women during the antepartum intrapartum period. Some of these women may benefit from a planned Caesarean section if they have had previous surgery breaching the uterine cavity or in cases of malpresentation. Women with known CUAs all need to also have their renal tract investigated either pre-pregnancy, antenatally or post-natally due to the high risk of associated renal anomalies.

The literature is still scant in terms of best evidence and more robust future research is required to ensure the effect of CUAs on pregnancy and obstetric outcomes is thoroughly investigated through well designed studies while considering potential confounders. This is so that we can optimise the care of these women through their pregnancy journey.

Clinical Governance Issues

- CUA have a 25% risk of concomitant renal tract anomalies and hence renal tract imaging is recommended if not done prior to pregnancy [4]
- A septate uterus is associated with the worst reproductive outcomes amongst CUAs with a live term birth rate of around 30% an increased risk of first trimester miscarriage, preterm birth, fetal growth restriction and fetal malpresentation at delivery
- An arcuate uterus may increase the risk of second trimester miscarriages and fetal malpresentation at birth
- Unification defects (unicornuate, bicornuate or didelphys uteri) significantly increase the risk of first trimester miscarriage, preterm birth, fetal malpresentation at delivery, low birth weight and pre-eclampsia. In those women, we would recommend appropriate preterm birth surveillance as well as fetal serial growth scanning
- Women with a rudimentary horn can sometimes present with a pregnancy in the horn, thereby increasing the risk of uterine rupture especially if it remains undiagnosed. If the rudimentary horn has a functioning endometrium, these women may benefit from laparoscopic excision of the horn
- Adequate and timely surgical excision of obstructing transverse septae is important to reduce morbidity but the location of the septum also affects the chance of conception with a high septum having the worst reproductive outcome
- In pregnant women with previous transverse septum, there is a risk of vaginal soft tissue dystocia during labour requiring an emergency Caesarean section or the risk of lacerations
- Excision of a longitudinal obstructing vaginal septae can improve the conception rate in women

- Controlled studies have shown that hysteroscopic resection of a uterine septum can reduce miscarriage rates and can therefore be offered to women with recurrent miscarriages or infertility. There is no place currently for offering a hysteroscopic resection routinely to an asymptomatic woman

References

1 M. A. Akhtar, S. H. Saravelos, T. C. Li and K. Jayaprakasan (on behalf of the Royal College of Obstetricians and Gynaecologists). Reproductive implications and management of congenital uterine anomalies. Scientific Impact Paper No. 62. *British Journal of Obstetrics and Gynaecology*, **127** (2020), e1–e13.

2 Y. Y. Chan, K. Jayaprakasan, J. Zamora, et al. The prevalence of congenital uterine anomalies in unselected and high-risk populations: A systematic review. *Human Reproduction Update*, **17** (2011),761–71.

3 American Fertility Society. The AFS classification of adnexal adhesions, distal tubal occlusion, tubal occlusion secondary to tubal ligation, tubal pregnancies, Müllerian anomalies and intrauterine adhesions. *Fertility and Sterility*, **49** (1988), 944–55.

4 G. F. Grimbizis, S. Gordts, A. Di Spiezio Sardo, et al. The ESHRE/ESGE consensus on the classification of female genital tract congenital anomalies. *Human Reproduction*, **28** (2013), 2032–44.

5 S. H. Saravelos, K. A. Cocksedge and T. C. Li. Prevalence and diagnosis of congenital uterine anomalies in women with reproductive failure: A critical appraisal. *Human Reproduction Update*, **14** (2008), 415–29.

6 L. Marcal, M. A. Nothaft, F. Coelho, R. Volpato and R. Iyer. Müllerian duct anomalies: MR imaging. *Abdominal Imaging*, **36** (2011), 756–64.

7 K. Jayaprakasan, Y. Y. Chan, S. Sur, et al. Prevalence of uterine anomalies and their impact on early pregnancy in women conceiving after assisted reproduction

treatment. *Ultrasound in Obstetrics & Gynecology*, **37** (2011), 727–32.

8 G. F. Grimbizis, A. Di Spiezio Sardo, S. H. Saravelos, et al. The Thessaloniki ESHRE/ESGE consensus on diagnosis of female genital anomalies. *Human Reproduction*, **31** (2016), 2–7.

9 Practice Committee of the American Society for Reproductive Medicine. Uterine septum: A guideline. *Fertility and Sterility*, **106** (2016), 530–40.

10 A. Ludwin, W. P. Martins, C. O. Nastri, et al. Congenital Uterine Malformation by Experts (CUME): Better criteria for distinguishing between normal/arcuate and septate uterus? *Ultrasound in Obstetrics & Gynecology*, **51** (2018), 101–9.

11 J. Knez, E. Saridogan, T. Van Den Bosch, et al. ESHRE/ESGE female genital tract anomalies classification system—the potential impact of discarding arcuate uterus on clinical practice. *Human Reproduction*, **33** (2018), 600–6.

12 B. W. Rackow and A. Arici. Reproductive performance of women with Müllerian anomalies. *Current Opinion in Obstetrics and Gynecology*, **19** (2007), 229–37.

13 Y. Y. Chan, K. Jayaprakasan, A. Tan, et al. Reproductive outcomes in women with congenital uterine anomalies: A systematic review. *Ultrasound in Obstetrics and Gynecology*, **38** (2011), 371–82.

14 C. A. Venetis, S. P. Papadopoulos, R. Campo, et al. Clinical implications of congenital uterine anomalies: A meta-analysis of comparative studies. *Reproductive BioMedicine Online*, **29** (2014), 665–83.

15 J. F. W. Rikken, C. R. Kowalik, M. H. Emanuel, et al. Septum resection for

women of reproductive age with a septate uterus. *Cochrane Database of Systematic Reviews*, **1** (2017), Art. No.:CD008576.

16 National Institute for Health and Care Excellence. *Hysteroscopic Metroplasty of a Uterine Septum for Recurrent Miscarriage.* NICE Interventional Procedures Guidance **510**. (London: NICE, 2015).

17 National Institute for Health and Care Excellence. *Hysteroscopic Metroplasty of a Uterine Septum for Primary Infertility.* NICE Interventional Procedures Guidance **509**. (London: NICE, 2015).

18 P. K. Heinonen. Distribution of female genital tract anomalies in two classifications. *European Journal of Obstetrics & Gynecology and Reproductive Biology*, **206** (2016), 141–6.

19 N. S. Fox, A. S. Roman, E. M. Stern, et al. Type of congenital uterine anomaly and adverse pregnancy outcomes. *Journal of Maternal-Fetal and Neonatal Medicine*, **27** (2014), 949–53.

20 G. G. Nahum. Rudimentary uterine horn pregnancy. The 20th century worldwide experience of 588 cases. *Journal of Reproductive Medicine*, **47** (2002), 151–63.

21 J. A. Rock, H. A. Zacur, A. M. Dlugi AM, et al. Pregnancy success following surgical correction of imperforate hymen and complete transverse vaginal septum. *Obstetrics & Gynecology*, **59** (1982), 448.

22 M. M. Joki-Erkkila and P. K. Heinonen. Presenting and long-term clinical implications and fecundity in females with obstructing vaginal malformations. *Journal of Pediatric and Adolescent Gynecology*, **16** (2003), 307–12.

23 C. E. Williams, R. S. Nakhal, M. A. Hall-Craggs, et al. Transverse vaginal septae: Management and long-term outcomes. *BJOG: An International Journal of Obstetrics & Gynaecology*, **121** (2014), 1653–8.

24 E. K. Saks, B. Vakili and A. C. Steinberg. Primary amenorrhoea with an abdominal mass at the umbilicus. *Journal of Pediatric and Adolescent Gynecology*, **22** (2009), e1–3.

25 G. B. Candiani, L. Fedele and M. Candiani. Double uterus, blind hemivagina, and ipsilateral renal agenesis: 36 cases and long-term follow-up. *Obstetrics & Gynecology*, **90** (1997), 26.

26 J. A. Rock and H. W. Jones. The double uterus associated with an obstructed hemivagina and ipsilateral renal agenesis. *American Journal of Obstetrics and Gynecology*, **138** (1980), 339–42.

27 B. Haddad, E. Barranger and B. J. Paniel. Blind hemivagina: Long-term follow-up and reproductive performance in 42 cases. *Human Reproduction*, **14** (1999), 1962.

28 D. L. Olive and D. Y. Henderson. Endometriosis and Müllerian anomalies. *Obstetrics & Gynecology*, **69** (1987), 412–15.

29. E. E. Wallach, J. A. Rock and W. D. Schlaff. The obstetric consequences of uterovaginal anomalies. *Fertility and Sterility*, **43** (1985), 681–92.

30 G. S. Letterie. Management of congenital uterine abnormalities. *Reproductive BioMedicine Online*, **23** (2011), 40–52.

31 G. B. Candiani, P. Vercellini, L. Fedele, et al. Repair of the uterine cavity after hysteroscopic septal incision. *Fertility and Sterility*, **54** (1990), 991–4.

32 J. H. Yang, M. J. Chen, C. D. Chen, et al. Optimal waiting period for subsequent fertility treatment after various hysteroscopic surgeries. *Fertility and Sterility*, **99** (2013), 2092–6.

Vaginal Prolapse and Previous Prolapse Surgery

6

Swati Jha

6.1 Introduction

Pelvic organ prolapse (POP) is a common condition affecting up to 50% of parous women, with documented evidence suggesting that approximately 11% of women will require a single operation for POP and urinary incontinence during their lifetime [1].

The aetiology of POP is complex and multifactorial. It is generally accepted that pregnancy and parturition play a significant role, since any structural damage to the anatomical supports of the pelvic organs, incorporating musculature, connective tissue and their associated nerve supplies, can be detrimental. Given that nulliparous women may also develop POP [2], childbirth is not exclusive to the development of POP. Vaginal delivery may result in pelvic support defects[3]. A study by Gyhagen et al. found that the prevalence of symptomatic POP was doubled after vaginal delivery compared with Caesarean section (CS), two decades after one birth [4]. This was irrespective of whether the Caesarean was elective or as an emergency [4]. With evidence emerging from imaging studies of the pelvic floor by Delancey [5–7], evidence of the role of instrumental deliveries in the development of prolapse is fast becoming obvious.

Mant et al. [8] reported that women with more than two vaginal deliveries have a four times greater risk of prolapse compared to nulliparous women.

Common risk factors for the development of POP include increasing age, parity and patient weight. Infant birth weight and current body mass index (BMI) are risk factors for POP after vaginal delivery [4]. Other risk factors include: congenital or acquired connective tissue disorders, race, raised intra-abdominal pressure, chronic disease and iatrogenic factors [4, 9]. Pregnancy itself as an isolated entity presents unique physiological risk factors for the development of POP, namely hormonal increases, such as cortisol, progesterone and relaxin, which can lead to a concomitant stretching of the pelvic structures. In addition, any structural changes as a result of the gravid uterus, cervical elongation and parturition can stretch tissues beyond their physiological limits and contribute to the development of POP during and after pregnancy. Glazener et al. in their 12 year longitudinal cohort have shown that women were more likely to have prolapse if they were older when they had their first baby, had more than one baby and if all their deliveries were spontaneous vaginal deliveries [10].

Prolapse may therefore be a symptom reported in parous women as a pre-existing condition. Mild POP that exists before pregnancy usually resolves spontaneously by the end of the second trimester [11]. Comparatively, the development of POP for the first time during pregnancy is rare, affecting one per 10, 000 to 15, 000 deliveries [12]. This can present at any stage of the pregnancy but usually in the first or second trimesters.

Women with prolapse either predating or presenting for the first time during pregnancy pose a clinical dilemma. The occurrence of POP in pregnancy has been extensively reported but the evidence for mode of delivery is limited.

With the rise of the average maternal age and BMI in today's antenatal population, POP during pregnancy remains a condition that every obstetrician should be familiar with managing as it poses several management dilemmas.

In this chapter, we will assess the current evidence base for the management of POP and women with previous prolapse surgery in the antenatal, intrapartum and post-partum periods and its associated complications as well as recommendations for delivery.

6.2 Antenatal

6.2.1 Women with Pre-existing Prolapse or First Presentation in Pregnancy

Women with pre-existing prolapse or development of POP for the first time in the antenatal period can present several problems for the attending obstetrician, depending on the extent of the prolapse and the symptoms experienced by the patient. Common symptoms include those experienced by non-pregnant women with prolapse and include the awareness of a vaginal lump, genital discomfort, backache, and difficulty voiding or defecating. In more severe cases women may present with urinary retention, cervical ulceration / bleeding, and preterm labour or miscarriage. A study in 2002 by Sze et al. demonstrated that in a cohort of 94 nulliparous patients, 46% (n = 43) developed a degree of POP by 36 weeks gestation, with 26% (n = 24) having a stage 2 prolapse noted (i.e. the most distal portion of the prolapse being 1 cm or less proximal or distal to the hymenal plane) [13]. This would suggest that simply carrying a pregnancy puts considerable strain on the pelvic floor resulting in a small prolapse, but whereas for some women this will resolve post-pregnancy, in others it will progress.

The management of POP antenatally is mainly conservative, aimed at symptomatic relief and there has been little change in this over the last century. Initial management, as documented by several reported cases is genital hygiene, followed by a period of rest. In cases of uterine/cervical prolapse, this may need to be in the Trendelenburg position to provide a degree of protection from injury and desiccation [14]. These initial conservative measures are often combined with generalised lifestyle advice, for example; smoking cessation, avoidance of heavy lifting, treating chronic cough, treating constipation and Kegal exercises[15].While there is some evidence to show that antenatal pelvic floor muscle training reduces post-partum stress urinary incontinence, the evidence for prevention of POP does not show the same effectiveness [16].

In order to provide continued support to the pelvic organs and alleviate prolapse symptoms, several authors have recommended the use of vaginal rings and pessaries. These rubber/silicone devices have widespread evidence of effectiveness for the management of POP in the non-pregnant population, especially when surgical measures are contraindicated or declined by patients. The non-invasive nature of a pessary means that it can be inserted and changed without risk to the patient or the pregnancy. Different pessaries used in the management of prolapse presenting in pregnancy are detailed in Table 6.1.

Piver et al. [17] reported a case series of eight patients experiencing uterine prolapse and recommend the use of a doughnut pessary to replace the prolapse and protect the

Table 6.1 Types of pessaries and their uses

Type of pessary	Image	Mechanism of action	Indication
Ring		Lodges between posterior fornix and pubic symphysis and replaces displaced uterus	All grades of uterovaginal prolapse
Hodge–Smith		Broad limb prevents pessary from turning in the vagina and keeps uterus anteverted	Uterine prolapse with retroverted uterus or urinary retention
Cube		Suction mechanism of the sides allows it to attach to the vaginal walls and occludes vagina	All grades of prolapse
Gellhorn		Lies behind the pubic symphysis and expands forming suction and rests against the leading edge of prolapse	All grades of prolapse
Doughnut		Occludes upper vagina	All grades of prolapse
Shelf pessary		Occludes upper vagina	All grades of prolapse

Table 6.1 (*cont.*)

Type of pessary	Image	Mechanism of action	Indication
Inflatable pessary		Occludes upper vagina. It is a doughnut which can be expanded	All grades of prolapse

cervix from the trauma of protrusion by occluding the upper vagina. The authors recommend leaving the pessary *in situ* until the onset of labour except for periodic cleaning. The frequency of changing the pessary in the antenatal period is reliant on the type of pessary, however, it should not be left in longer than six months. If the same pessary is being reused, it should be cleaned with a mild soapy solution before reinsertion. Sawyer et al. [18] recommended the use of a Hodge–Smith pessary to restore a uterine prolapse antenatally until delivery. This pessary is less likely to turn or place undue pressure on the urethra. In contrast Yogev et al. [19] trialled the ring pessary in their case series; however, they noted displacement of the pessary, which fell out a few days after insertion. The same outcome occurred following the use of a Mayer's (Dumontpallier's) pessary by Horowitz et al. (11). The Gellhorn pessary has also been used for antenatal prolapse reduction with success [14]. This pessary produces a suction effect which aids placement; however, it can also mean that it is more difficult to remove. Cube pessaries and inflatable doughnuts have also been described for use in pregnancy related POP. Given the lack of consensus, it is sensible to use the ring in the first instance and if this fails then to consider alternatives.

Surgical correction of POP during pregnancy is not routinely undertaken, primarily due to the possible risks to both mother and fetus, but also as the long-term consequences are unknown. Matsumoto et al. [20] report a single case of entire uterine prolapse in a parous patient at 12 weeks gestation, where conservative measures were not effective. They performed a modified laparoscopic Gilliam uterine suspension procedure, whereby the round ligaments were fixed bilaterally to the rectus fascia with the aid of silicon sheets. The patient went on to have a spontaneous vaginal delivery at term with no complications of prolapse.

6.2.2 Women with Previous Prolapse Surgery

Women who become pregnant after POP surgery present a new conundrum to the obstetrician, since it is unknown what the effect of the pregnancy will be on the surgically corrected pelvic floor. There appears to be some evidence for this based on a study looking at Hospital Episode Statistics in England, 2002–2008, which showed that the incidence of further pelvic floor surgery after childbirth was lower after Caesarean delivery than after vaginal delivery, and this may indicate a protective effect of abdominal delivery [21]. There is limited evidence on the optimal route of delivery in women who have had previous prolapse surgery. Women presenting with prolapse should always be advised by their gynaecologist that surgery should be delayed till after childbearing is complete due to the risk of recurrence of POP and possible need for CS. However, because younger women are coming forwards for POP surgery and women are having babies later in life, it is inevitable that more women will present in pregnancy following POP surgery. In addition, women are choosing uterine preserving options for treatment which means they may find themselves pregnant accidentally, though some will plan this. For accidental pregnancies, women will sometimes choose to terminate due to the risk of recurrence, but some women will choose to continue the pregnancy [22].

The antenatal care of these women is as standard for any parturient. They need to be informed of the risk of recurrence during the antenatal period and a discussion about the mode of delivery is important. Unfortunately, there is no consensus on the optimal mode of delivery and recurrences have been seen both after CS as well as after a vaginal delivery. Women should be informed that the risk of recurrence appears to be higher following a vaginal delivery than after a CS based on the limited available evidence [21]. In some scenarios, a vaginal delivery may not actually be an option as the mesh used for correction of their prolapse intra- abdominally can be wrapped around the cervix, which would prevent the cervix from dilating if a woman was to go into labour.

There may also be safety concerns from the use of mesh for POP surgery in the antenatal period. The use of a sacrohysteropexy mesh has the potential risk of restricting uterine changes needed to support fetal growth and may require growth scans in the antenatal period. In addition, the posterior arms of the mesh have been reported to cause pain [23, 24], which may be relieved by the use of a pessary. A Manchester repair on the other hand is associated with a high risk of spontaneous miscarriage and preterm delivery [25]. Cervical length monitoring in women who are pregnant following a Manchester repair has not been widely studied, but it may be worth considering. Interpretation however is likely to be difficult.

There has only been one case to date of a pregnancy following a vaginal mesh implant and no obstetric complications were noted during pregnancy [26].

6.3 Intrapartum

6.3.1 Women with Pre-existing Prolapse or First Presentation in Pregnancy

The majority of patients with a minor degree of POP will go on to deliver spontaneously at term without any sequelae [17]. However, those patients with significant POP, especially where there is severe uterine or cervical descent may experience a high-risk labour and delivery. There are reports of stillbirth with a severe POP [27, 28]; however, these are few and most pregnancies result in live-birth pregnancies. It is also difficult to establish whether the stillbirth was caused by the prolapse or unrelated reasons.

When looking at the mode of delivery, the cases that report a CS are usually those presenting prematurely with severe prolapse needing delivery due to obstetric reasons [29] or extreme uterine descent [30], or patients in whom surgical correction of the prolapse was planned at the time of the delivery such as a CS hysterectomy [31] with attachment of the vault to the sacrum or an abdominal hysteropexy [32]. In most cases at term a CS seems to be avoidable with a Dührssen's incision, should the cervix fail to dilate.

Intrapartum complications from uterine or cervical POP include failure to progress, cervical dystocia as a result of oedema of the cervix, cervical lacerations and obstructive labour with an increased risk of uterine rupture [14, 33]. Historically, concerns over cervical dystocia often resulted in procedures to incise the cervix to facilitate dilatation and prevent overstretching of the lower uterine segment, such as Dührssen's incisions as recommended by Piver et al. [17]. The largest series on prolapse in pregnancy by Pandey et al. [34] report on frequent performance of Dührssen's incisions to avoid a CS, which has also been reported in other series [35]. An article by Lau et al. in 2008 suggests that cervical oedema can be overcome by topical application of a magnesium sulphate solution to the cervix in order to prevent cervical dystocia and lacerations [36]. Caesarean delivery however still remains a favoured choice amongst several authors for those women at high risk in labour from the complications of POP [19, 37–39] but there seems to be little evidence for this as complications with vaginal delivery in women with prolapse are rare and difficult to predict.

If a vaginal delivery is achieved then the birth attendant should be vigilant and monitor for primary post-partum haemorrhage, as both an over stretched lower uterine segment and cervical oedema can predispose to an atonic haemorrhage.

6.3.2 Women with Previous Prolapse Surgery

The majority of obstetricians would err on the side of caution and offer an elective CS in an attempt to protect against further *de novo* prolapse [15]. There are no Royal College of Obstetricians and Gynaecologists (RCOG) guidelines on optimal mode of delivery for this cohort of patients. The American Urogynaecological Society (AUGS) have issued recommendations on mode of delivery in women who have had previous surgery for POP, which may be a guide [40].

Usually, these women undergo an elective CS to avoid the risk of recurrence of prolapse. However, a CS is not necessarily protective and there are cases reported of recurrence even after a CS [24]. It is important to remember that most case series and studies only follow women up for a finite period of time so it is difficult to know what proportion of women who have had a CS to prevent recurrence of prolapse go on to have a POP again in later life.

Following a sacrohysteropexy [22–24] it would be usual to perform a CS, and in the single reported case of pregnancy following a transvaginal mesh the delivery was also by CS [26].

The reported cases of delivery following a uterosacral ligament hysteropexy were all by CS [41, 42]. However, following a sacrospinous hysteropexy, both vaginal delivery and CS have been reported with variable outcomes [43, 44]. Following a Manchester repair, though, there are no contraindications to a vaginal delivery, labour dystocia may occur as well as preterm labour.

Because of limited data it is difficult to make clear recommendations regarding the mode of delivery following individual procedures such as anterior and posterior vaginal wall repairs.

6.4 Post-Partum

Interestingly, though pelvic floor muscle training (PFMT) is routinely advised to women post-natally to prevent prolapse, Bo et al. [45] in a recent study failed to show a difference of post-partum PFMT on POP in primiparous women. More randomised control trials (RCTs) are needed before strong conclusions can be drawn in this particular population.

POP if present antenatally will usually persist or recur after delivery [14]. Additionally, a new POP can occur and be symptomatic during the puerperium. Sze et al. [13] found that 13/41 women (32%) who had spontaneous vaginal delivery and 9/26 (35%) who had Caesarean delivery during active labour developed a new prolapse by six weeks post-natally.

Continued conservative treatment measures should be employed to manage POP post-natally, especially if the woman has not yet completed her family. They should be advised that surgery carries the risk of requiring a CS in a future pregnancy. For women who wish to discuss their options, a referral to a urogynaecologist should be considered. If surgical measures are to be considered to correct POP post-natally, then there are a lack of data pertaining to the ideal time interval between delivery and subsequent surgical management. However, logic would dictate that there be at least a three-month interval between delivery and surgical correction to allow the physiological changes of pregnancy to return to the pre-pregnancy state.

The choice of surgical procedure for POP is dependent on whether the woman wants to preserve her fertility. In general, women with POP who wish to preserve their fertility should be offered conservative management in the first instance [15]. Failure of conservative measures may result in surgical options being considered and a variety of fertility-sparing procedures have been described. Results for efficacy and subsequent fertility rates are however limited. These procedures can include open or laparoscopic uterine suspension procedures, uterosacral suspension and sacrospinous uterine fixation [46, 47]. Maher et al. report a case series of 43 women who underwent laparoscopic suture hysteropexy [42]. From their cohort, two women achieved term pregnancies delivered by elective CS. Seracchioli et al. report a case series of 15 women who underwent a conservative laparoscopic surgical correction of genital prolapse and noted that three became pregnant, culminating in two term Caesarean deliveries and one eight-week abortion [48].

6.5 Clinical Dilemmas

Nulliparous women planning a single pregnancy may be advised that vaginal delivery compared with CS carries a greater risk of symptomatic POP (14.6 versus 6.3%, odds ratio [OR] 2.55) [4]. Women who deliver all babies by CS also seem to experience a protective effect [10]. The results of the Swedish Pregnancy, Obesity and Pelvic Floor (SWEPOP) study indicate that 12 CSs need to be performed to avoid one case of symptomatic POP [4]. However, in this study, in those women of short stature (<160 cm), with an infant weighing more than 4000 g the 'number needed to treat' was only two. This suggests that in these at-risk patients a CS might be preventative. These results apply to women who have no pre-existing POP. Additionally, in women planning one or two children, elective CS may be considered depending on individual preferences, requests and after appropriate counselling. However, the long-term impact of exclusive CS is yet to be seen.

Women with various grades of existing prolapse who become pregnant are often anxious to avoid delivery vaginally and will often request a CS to prevent worsening of the prolapse. They are usually parous women who have had previous vaginal deliveries. Counselling is more difficult as evidence is limited. The study by Glazener et al. suggests that women with mixed spontaneous vaginal delivery and CS may be less likely to have prolapse, however, the mean population of their cohort was relatively young (i.e. 42 years) [10]. This is significantly younger than women who normally seek surgical correction of their prolapse. In addition, this is based on the findings of 59 women, hence numbers are too small to draw meaningful conclusions [10]. The authors add that the findings of that study are at odds with each other, and further follow-up is required [10]. Hence, when counselling women with prolapse in pregnancy or preceding the pregnancy, it needs to be emphasised that there is no evidence that delivering by CS alters the long-term outcome and there is insufficient evidence to suggest proven benefit. The same is applicable to women who present with prolapse in their first pregnancy.

6.6 Conclusion

Although rare, POP complicating a pregnancy can be fraught with significant problems both mentally and physically for the woman. The impact of elective Caesarean delivery in women who have a prolapse presenting in pregnancy is poorly understood. Exclusive Caesarean delivery may be a preventative strategy against POP, but this needs to be weighed up against the risks associated with repeat Caesarean delivery. Symptomatic correction remains the mainstay of treatment and this has been the case over the last century, employing conservative techniques to temporarily support the pelvic organs during the pregnancy. This is usually achieved with bed rest, though a significant proportion of women will need a pessary for symptom control. Often the need for a ring is obviated by the middle of the second trimester. Obstetricians need to be aware of the different types of pessaries available for the management of POP as the traditional ring pessaries may not work. The mode of delivery is usually vaginal, however, awareness of features such as cervical inflammation and oedema should raise alertness to the possibility of dystocia, lacerations and tears, and lower the threshold for a Caesarean delivery. Post-natally, the patient must be cautioned of the probability of prolapse recurrence. Definitive surgical correction should be delayed by at least three months and longer if the patient is breastfeeding, to allow the physiological changes of pregnancy to settle. However, due to limited numbers and difficulty in establishing long-term outcomes there are obvious problems in conducting RCTs to address this issue. We are therefore reliant on observational studies to provide much needed answers to a common but pressing clinical problem and more research is needed into the management of women presenting in pregnancy with prolapse.

Clinical Governance Issues
- Women with pre-existing POP should be advised on conservative treatment strategies during pregnancy. Where bothersome, a pessary should be considered
- Women who have already had a vaginal delivery and are worried about worsening of prolapse should be advised that subsequent CS is unlikely to be protective as the damage to the pelvic floor has already occurred
- Clinicians should be aware of the intrapartum risks of cervical dystocia and post-partum haemorrhage in women going into labour with a uterine prolapse and should be alert to these to facilitate prompt management
- Women of short stature with a large baby are at significantly increased risk of POP and a discussion about family size and mode of delivery should take place antenatally

- Women should be advised to delay surgery for POP till after childbearing is complete
- When women require surgery for POP post-natally this should be delayed till after three months or cessation of breastfeeding with advice about PFMT in the interim and use of pessaries where needed
- Women unsure whether their family is complete and wishing surgical correction of POP should be advised they may need a CS if they have a pregnancy after their POP surgery. There is still a risk of recurrence even if they have a CS
- If every woman were to have exclusive CS for delivery, 12 CS would be required to prevent one case of POP as many other factors contribute
- Women should be informed that a forceps delivery increases the risk of POP

References

1 C. C. Liang, L. H. Tseng, S. G. Horng, I. W. Lin and S. D. Chang. Correlation of pelvic organ prolapse quantification system scores with obstetric parameters and lower urinary tract symptoms in primiparae postpartum. *International Urogynecology Journal and Pelvic Floor Dysfunction,* **18** (2007), 537–41.

2 H. Ishida, K. Takahashi and H. Kurachi. Uterine prolapse during late pregnancy in a nulliparous woman. *International Urogynecology Journal,* **25** (2014), 1739–40.

3 A. L. O'Boyle, P. J. Woodman, J. D. O'Boyle, G. D. Davis and S. E. Swift. Pelvic organ support in nulliparous pregnant and nonpregnant women: A case control study. *American Journal of Obstetrics and Gynecology,* **187** (2002), 99–102.

4 M. Gyhagen, M. Bullarbo, T. F. Nielsen and I. Milsom. Prevalence and risk factors for pelvic organ prolapse 20 years after childbirth: A national cohort study in singleton primiparae after vaginal or caesarean delivery. *British Journal of Obstetrics & Gynaecology,* **120** (2013), 152–60.

5 J. O. DeLancey, D. M. Morgan, D. E. Fenner, et al. Comparison of levator ani muscle defects and function in women with and without pelvic organ prolapse. *Obstetrics & Gynecology,* **109** (2007), 295–302.

6 R. Kearney, J. M. Miller, J. A. Ashton-Miller and J. O. DeLancey. Obstetric factors associated with levator ani muscle injury after vaginal birth. *Obstetrics & Gynecology,* **107** (2006), 144–9.

7 R. Kearney, M. Fitzpatrick, S. Brennan, et al. Levator ani injury in primiparous women with forceps delivery for fetal distress, forceps for second stage arrest, and spontaneous delivery. *International Journal of Gynaecology and Obstetrics,* **111** (2010), 19–22.

8 J. Mant, R. Painter and M. Vessey. Epidemiology of genital prolapse: Observations from the Oxford Family Planning Association Study. *British Journal of Obstetrics and Gynaecology,* **104** (1997), 579–85.

9 I. Nygaard, C. Bradley and D. Brandt. Pelvic organ prolapse in older women: Prevalence and risk factors. *Obstetrics & Gynecology,* **104**, (2004), 489–97.

10 C. Glazener, A. Elders, C. Macarthur, et al. Childbirth and prolapse: Long-term associations with the symptoms and objective measurement of pelvic organ prolapse. *British Journal of Obstetrics and Gynaecology,* **120** (2013),161–8.

11 E. R. Horowitz, Y. Yogev, M. Hod and B. Kaplan. Prolapse and elongation of the cervix during pregnancy. *International Journal of Gynaecology and Obstetrics,* **77** (2002), 147–8.

12 W. C. Keettel. Prolapse of uterus during pregnancy. *American Journal of Obstetrics and Gynecology,* **42** (1941), 21–6.

13 E. H. Sze, G. B. Sherard III and J. M. Dolezal. Pregnancy, labor, delivery, and pelvic organ prolapse. *Obstetrics & Gynecology*, **100** (2002), 981–6.

14 N. Mohamed-Suphan and R. K. Ng. Uterine prolapse complicating pregnancy and labor: A case report and literature review. *International Urogynecology Journal*, **23** (2012), 647–50.

15 F. Asali, I. Mahfouz and C. Phillips. The management of urogynaecological problems in pregnancy and the early postpartum period. *Obstetrics & Gynecology*, **14** (2012), 153–8.

16 K. E. Romeikiene and D. Bartkeviciene. Pelvic-floor dysfunction prevention in prepartum and postpartum periods. *Medicina (Kaunas)*, **57** (2021), 387.

17 M. S. Piver and J. Spezia. Uterine prolapse during pregnancy. *Obstetrics & Gynecology*, **32** (1968), 765–9.

18 D. Sawyer and K. Frey. Cervical prolapse during pregnancy. *Journal of the American Board of Family Practice*, **13** (2000), 216–18.

19 Y. Yogev, E. R. Horowitz, A. Ben Haroush and B. Kaplan. Uterine cervical elongation and prolapse during pregnancy: An old unsolved problem. *Clinical and Experimental Obstetrics & Gynecology*, **30** (2003), 183–5.

20 T. Matsumoto, M. Nishi, M. Yokota and M. Ito. Laparoscopic treatment of uterine prolapse during pregnancy. *Obstetrics & Gynecology*, **93** (1999), 849.

21 A. Pradhan, D. G. Tincello and R. Kearney. Childbirth after pelvic floor surgery: Analysis of Hospital Episode Statistics in England, 2002–2008. *British Journal of Obstetrics and Gynaecology*, **120** (2013), 200–4.

22 E. Barranger, X. Fritel and A. Pigne. Abdominal sacrohysteropexy in young women with uterovaginal prolapse: Long-term follow-up. *American Journal of Obstetrics and Gynecology*, **189** (2003), 1245–50.

23 G. Busby and J. Broome. Successful pregnancy outcome following laparoscopic sacrohysteropexy for second degree uterine prolapse. *Gynecological Surgery*, **7** (2010), 271–3.

24 C. M. Lewis and P. Culligan. Sacrohysteropexy followed by successful pregnancy and eventual reoperation for prolapse. *International Urogynecology Journal*, **23** (2012), 957–9.

25 J. J. Fisher. The effect of amputation of the cervix uteri upon subsequent parturition: A preliminary report of seven cases. *American Journal of Obstetrics and Gynecology*, **62** (1951), 644–8.

26 Y. Kumtepe, K. Cetinkaya and Y. Karasu. Pregnancy and delivery after anterior vaginal mesh replacement: A case presentation. *International Urogynecology Journal*, **24** (2013), 345–7.

27 S. Pantha. Repeated pregnancy in a woman with uterine prolapse from a rural area in Nepal. *Reproductive Health Matters*, **19** (2011), 129–32.

28 S. Yousaf, B. Haq and T. Rana. Extensive uterovaginal prolapse during labor. *Journal of Obstetrics and Gynaecology Research*, **37** (2011), 264–6.

29 G. A. Partsinevelos, S. Mesogitis, N. Papantoniou and A. Antsaklis. Uterine prolapse in pregnancy: A rare condition an obstetrician should be familiar with. *Fetal Diagnosis and Therapy*, **24** (2008), 296–8.

30 B. Cingillioglu, M. Kulhan and Y. Yildirim. Extensive uterine prolapse during active labor: A case report. *International Urogynecology Journal*, **21** (2010), 1433–4.

31 M. M. Meydanli, Y. Ustun and O. T. Yalcin. Pelvic organ prolapse complicating third trimester pregnancy. A case report. *Gynecologic and Obstetric Investigation*, **61** (2006), 133–4.

32 R. Karatayli, K. Gezginc, A. H. Kantarci and A. Acar. Successful treatment of uterine prolapse by abdominal hysteropexy performed during Cesarean section. *Archives of Gynecology and Obstetrics*, **287** (2013), 319–22.

33 L. Guariglia, B. Carducci, A. Botta, S. Ferrazzani and A. Caruso. Uterine

prolapse in pregnancy. *Gynecologic and Obstetric Investigation*, **60** (2005), 192–4.

34 K. Pandey, S. Arya and S. Pande. Pregnancy with uterine prolapse: Dührssen's incision still valid in today's scenario? *International Journal of Reproduction, Contraception, Obstetrics and Gynecology*, **2** (2013), 586–90.

35 H. L. Brown. Cervical prolapse complicating pregnancy. *Journal of the National Medical Association*, **89** (1997), 346–8.

36 S. Lau and A. Rijhsinghani. Extensive cervical prolapse during labor: A case report. *Journal of Reproductive Medicine*, **53** (2008), 67–9.

37 C. Kart, T. Aran and S. Guven. Stage IV C prolapse in pregnancy. *International Journal of Gynaecology & Obstetrics*, **112** (2011), 142–3.

38 S. Chandru, J. Srinivasan and A. D. Roberts. Acute uterine cervical prolapse in pregnancy. *Journal of Obstetrics and Gynaecology*, **27** (2007), 423–4.

39 G. Daskalakis, E. Lymberopoulos, E. Anastasakis, et al. Uterine prolapse complicating pregnancy. *Archives of Gynecology and Obstetrics*, **276** (2007), 391–2.

40 C. K. Wieslander, M. M. Weinstein, V. L. Handa and S. A. Collins. Pregnancy in women with prior treatments for pelvic floor disorders. *Female Pelvic Medicine and Reconstructive Surgery*, **26** (2020), 299–305.

41 N. Kow, H. B. Goldman and B. Ridgeway. Uterine conservation during prolapse repair: 9-year experience at a single institution. *Female Pelvic Medicine and Reconstructive Surgery*, **22** (2016), 126–31.

42 C. F. Maher, M. P. Carey and C. J. Murray. Laparoscopic suture hysteropexy for uterine prolapse. *Obstetrics and Gynecology*, **97** (2001), 1010–14.

43 M. Hefni and T. El-Toukhy. Sacrospinous cervico-colpopexy with follow-up 2 years after successful pregnancy. *European Journal of Obstetrics & Gynecology and Reproductive Biology*, **103** (2002), 188–90.

44 S. R. Kovac and S. H. Cruikshank. Successful pregnancies and vaginal deliveries after sacrospinous uterosacral fixation in five of nineteen patients. *American Journal of Obstetrics and Gynecology*, **168** (1993), 1778–83.

45 K. Bo, G. Hilde, J. Staer-Jensen, et al. Postpartum pelvic floor muscle training and pelvic organ prolapse. *American Journal of Obstetrics and Gynecology*, **212** (2015), e1–7.

46 L. L. Lin, M. H. Ho, A. L. Haessler, et al. A review of laparoscopic uterine suspension procedures for uterine preservation. *Current Opinion in Obstetrics and Gynecology*, **17** (2005), 541–6.

47 A. Cutner, R. Kearney and A. Vashisht. Laparoscopic uterine sling suspension: A new technique of uterine suspension in women desiring surgical management of uterine prolapse with uterine conservation. *British Journal of Obstetrics and Gynaecology*, **114** (2007), 1159–62.

48 R. Seracchioli, J. A. Hourcabie, F. Vianello, et al. Laparoscopic treatment of pelvic floor defects in women of reproductive age. *Journal of the American Association of Gynecologic Laparoscopists*, **11** (2004), 332–5.

Urinary Tract Problems
in Pregnancy

Neil Harvey, Ian Pearce, Rohna Kearney

7.1 Urinary Incontinence

Lower urinary tract symptoms are common during pregnancy with two thirds of women reporting urinary frequency and nocturia. It is important to rule out urine infection as a cause of urinary symptoms during pregnancy. Urinary incontinence (UI) can occur for the first time antenatally or women with pre-existing UI can experience worsening symptoms during pregnancy. A cohort study of 547 women recruited from a maternity clinic in a tertiary hospital in Finland reported a prevalence of UI during mid-pregnancy of 39% [1]. This study found that women who had UI before pregnancy and during pregnancy were more likely to report UI post-natally. A Taiwanese study of personal interviews of 270 women attending antenatal clinics reported a prevalence of urinary frequency in 77%, nocturia in 76%, stress urinary incontinence (SUI) in 51% and urgency urinary incontinence (UUI) in 10% [2]. Several studies have reported that women who have UI before and/or during pregnancy are more likely to have persistent UI after pregnancy [3, 4].

SUI is the complaint of any involuntary loss of urine on effort or physical exertion [5]. It is commonly reported in pregnant women. The main intervention to prevent and treat UI during pregnancy is supervised pelvic floor muscle training (PFMT). A Cochrane review reports that women performing antenatal PFMT probably have a lower risk of reporting UI in late pregnancy and that current evidence suggests that antenatal PFMT slightly decreases the risk of UI in the mid-post-natal period [6]. The review found no evidence that antenatal PFMT in incontinent women decreases UI in late pregnancy or in the post-natal period. In post-natal women with persistent UI, there is no evidence that PFMT results in a difference in UI at more than 6–12 months postpartum. The National Institute of Clinical Excellence (NICE) guidance on pelvic floor dysfunction recommends that women who are pregnant are encouraged to do PFMT and that a three-month programme of supervised PFMT should be considered from week 20 of pregnancy for pregnant women who have a first degree relative with pelvic floor dysfunction [7].

UUI is the complaint of involuntary loss of urine associated with urgency. Although less commonly reported in pregnancy than SUI, it is more commonly reported combined with symptoms of SUI and this is called mixed UI. Treatment is usually PFMT combined with lifestyle advice on stopping smoking, optimising weight and reducing caffeine intake. Pharmacotherapy for overactive bladder is not recommended during pregnancy or while breastfeeding.

7.1.1 Previous Surgery for Stress Urinary Incontinence

Most obstetricians recommend delivery by Caesarean section (CS) in women with a history of previous pelvic floor surgery to reduce the risk of recurrence of pelvic floor symptoms. There is very little evidence on the long-term outcome of women who deliver after a pelvic floor procedure. An analysis of Hospital Episode Statistics in England recorded 603 women who had a delivery episode after previous pelvic floor surgery between 2002–2008 [8]. In this group, 42 women had a further pelvic floor surgery episode following delivery in the same time period. The incidence of repeat surgery was higher in the group delivered vaginally than in those delivered by Caesarean (13.6 vs 4.4%). Fourteen of the 42 women had undergone previous surgery for incontinence prior to index delivery.

A register-based case-control study of women with a mid-urethral sling procedure for SUI in Finland reported 94 cases with a subsequent pregnancy and 330 controls without a subsequent pregnancy matched by age, operation type and year [9]. Over a follow-up of 10 years it found no difference in the number of SUI re-operations between cases and controls. The rate of vaginal delivery was 57% compared with 91% before the mid-urethral sling procedure.

7.2 Urinary Retention during Pregnancy and Post-Partum (URPP)

While the nomenclature for the two main categories of urinary retention differ between the urological and the obstetric literature, the terms are synonymous. Acute or overt urinary retention is defined as a generally (but not always) painful, palpable or percussable bladder, when the patient is unable to pass any urine when the bladder is full [5]. Classically, this is specifically a sudden onset of the inability to void [10]. Chronic/covert urinary retention is defined as a non-painful bladder, where there is a chronic high post-void residual. There remains disagreement over the definition of a high post-void residual, however. Obstetric literature and guidelines use a much higher threshold (of $\geq$150 ml after two or more voids) than urological literature where significance would be considered anything $\geq$50 ml [11, 12], accepting that residuals are commonly higher (i.e. $\geq$150 ml). The long-term harm of self-limiting peripartum chronic retention of urine remains to be demonstrated, and it is only significant as a risk factor for subsequent precipitation of peripartum acute urinary retention. Peripartum chronic retention can be expected to resolve over weeks post-partum.

In pregnancy, acute retention typically occurs between 14–16 weeks of pregnancy although it can occur at any stage. Chronic retention is usually only diagnosed incidentally during pregnancy or may have been present prior to pregnancy. There are several contributing risk factors for the development of urinary retention (Table 7.1).

7.2.1 Pathophysiology

The pathophysiology of URPP is multifactorial. The loss of detrusor muscle tone due to hormonal changes during pregnancy results in increased functional bladder capacity that usually goes unnoticed by the patient due to the increased uterine volume and associated increase in intra-abdominal pressure facilitating effective voiding. The intra-abdominal urethra elongates as part of the physiological response to pregnancy to reduce stress incontinence. Post-partum, the sudden loss of this increased abdominal pressure, coupled with post-partum diuresis, results in a low-pressure bladder that, when overdistended, is unable to mount an effective detrusor contraction necessary to void. Direct pressure of

Table 7.1 Risk factors for urinary retention can be divided into (pre-existing) gynaecological, obstetric and urological/other causes

Gynaecological	Obstetric	Urological/Other
Congenital uterine abnormalities	Anterior, complex or extensive vaginal/perineal perinatal haematoma/trauma	Constipation
History of female genital mutilation	Caesarean section (CS)	Macrosomia
Nulliparous/primigravida	Instrumental delivery	Need to catheterise in labour
Retroverted uterus	Manual delivery of placenta	Pre-existing urinary dysfunction – before or during pregnancy
Uterine fibroids	Prolonged labour, particularly active second stage	Significant immobility
	Regional anaesthesia	Urinary tract infection
	Significant oedema	

the presenting fetal head towards the end of pregnancy and during labour can obstruct the bladder outlet and contribute to a pelvic nerve neuropraxia, which can be compounded by labour and delivery. Lastly, perineal pain can contribute to failure of relaxation of the external urethral sphincter during voiding, which is more common after instrumental delivery or following significant perineal trauma.

7.2.2 Assessment and Management of URPP: Antenatal, Perinatal and Post-Partum

Internationally, it is recognised that there is a paucity of guidelines concerning the management of urinary retention during pregnancy [13]. The Institute of Obstetricians and Gynaecologists (Royal College of Physicians of Ireland) and the Directorate of Clinical Strategy and Programmes (Health Service Executive of Ireland) have jointly published the most extensive guidelines covering the management of urinary retention in pregnancy and post-partum [14].

The Royal College of Obstetricians and Gynaecologists last released guidelines, since retired, on the topic in 2002, and the National Institute for Health and Care Excellence (NICE) make only six recommendations regarding urine output:

1. Frequency of urination is recorded during the first stage of labour [15]
2. Frequency of urination is recorded during the second stage of labour [15]
3. Assess the patient for transfer to obstetric-led care if, after six hours, their bladder is palpable and they are unable to pass urine [15]
4. Insert a urethral catheter for 24 hours in cases of perineal repair [15]
5. Patients having a CS with regional anaesthesia should have an indwelling catheter to prevent-overdistension of the bladder, which can be removed after the patient is mobile, but no sooner than 12 hours after the last 'top-up' dose [16]
6. After CS, urinary retention should be considered in the differentials of severe pain unresponsive to analgesia and of urinary symptoms [16]

7.2.3 Antenatal Urinary Retention

Antenatal urinary retention is typically acute, with the patient presenting with pain-related distress. History taking should briefly cover the salient points of preceding urinary symptoms (including of urinary tract infection), fluid intake and preceding output times and volumes, and recent bowel habits (e.g. constipation). Examination can be limited to palpation of the bladder. Automated ultrasound bladder scanning can incorrectly recognise amniotic fluid as bladder volume and should be considered unreliable. Immediate management is transurethral catheterisation of the bladder, with as narrow a catheter as possible. Latex coated polytetrafluoroethylene catheters are softer, more comfortable and less likely to cause any subsequent issue with stricture disease. A 'male length'/longer catheter is safer due to elongation of the urethra. Any distress should settle rapidly. If the catheter even drains a small volume, and any pain has not settled, an alternative diagnosis is more likely than an incorrectly sited catheter.

In cases of indwelling catheterisation, a trial without catheter can be considered based on the following timeframe. If at the point of trial without catheter a patient is able to void more than >200 ml twice with normal bladder sensation and a residual volume <150 ml, then it is successful.

If unsuccessful, clean intermittent (self-)catheterisation (CIC) can be taught and subsequently ceased when residual volumes are <150 ml on two sequential occasions [14].

7.2.4 Peripartum Urinary Retention

Management is primarily focussed on early recognition, with patients being encouraged to void every four hours during labour and post-partum and voiding episodes recorded. If unable to void at four hours, conservative measures including privacy, analgesia, managing constipation if required, assistance with mobilisation and leaning forward to void or sitting in a warm bath/shower should all be offered. Patients unable to void by six hours or presenting with any of the other urinary storage symptoms should be offered catheterisation. For this initial occurrence either an indwelling 12Ch urethral catheter or CIC should be utilised. If four hours after a single CIC the patient is unable to void again, an indwelling catheter is more appropriate. It is critical that any indwelling catheter be removed (or at a minimum, any balloon deflated and the catheter taped to the patient's leg) prior to the active second stage of labour to prevent associated trauma to the urethra. Spinal anaesthesia is a significant risk factor for urinary retention and women receiving a spinal anaesthetic should routinely be catheterised.

7.2.5 Post-Partum Urinary Retention (PPUR)

The criteria for defining PPUR are as above, with persistent PPUR specifically used to describe retention lasting >72 hours. The most important aspects of management are again early recognition (with features outlined previously), and avoidance – particularly by following the above guidelines on minimum durations of catheterisation, and in addition, for at least six hours after an epidural (or until full bladder sensation returns if no other risk factors). For the patient who had a vaginal delivery without regional anaesthesia, if able to void >150 ml within four hours post-partum, there is little concern and no further action is needed. At four hours without voiding, the same conservative measures as in the peripartum urinary retention pathway should be

Table 7.2 Recommended duration of catheterisation by residual volume [14])

Residual volume after catheterisation	Duration of catheterisation
<150 ml	Catheter can be removed
>150–500 ml	24 hours
>500–1000 ml	48 hours
>1000 ml	72 hours

undertaken. If there is any concern whatsoever, residual volume must be determined by CIC and an indwelling catheter considered with residual volumes >150 ml.

The importance of good post-partum bladder management stems from the concern that if the bladder remains in a hyperdistended state post-partum for a protracted period it may ultimately result in an irreversible detrusor muscle injury. This may be either complete (acontractile bladder) or incomplete (detrusor underactivity), presenting as a slow urinary stream, hesitancy and straining to void, with or without a feeling of incomplete bladder emptying, sometimes with storage symptoms [17]. In cases of detrusor underactivity long-term, clean intermittent self-catheterisation is the mainstay of treatment. In situations where this is not feasible (or tolerated) urethrally, a continent cutaneous catheterisable channel (i.e. a Mitrofanoff) is the most appropriate next option in selected patients. The option of last resort is long-term catheterisation, with the suprapubic route preferred to negate the risk of later developing a patulous urethra, and to facilitate future catheter changes [18].

The significance of specific volumes of post-void residual urine and how this should factor into the duration of catheterisation is debated in the literature. The length of catheterisation may depend on how quickly perineal pain and discomfort resolves. An example system is set out in Table 7.2 [14]).

7.3 Urinary Diversions and Mitrofanoffs during Pregnancy

Urinary tract reconstruction involving the bowel includes numerous separate procedures including: continent and incontinent diversion using the small bowel, large bowel or a combination; augmentation of the bladder using the small bowel (or rarely other options, such as the stomach); and catheterisable conduits such as Mitrofanoff (appendicovesicostomy) and Monti (detubularised ileal segments) procedures. Urinary diversions primarily impact pregnancy and delivery in two ways: metabolic and surgical (i.e. CS).

In urinary pregnancy testing in cases of continent reservoirs and bladder augmentations, false positives occur due to mucous secreted by the bowel segment. If positive, confirmation is required with serum hCG testing before changing any clinical decision [19]. Exposure of the donor intestinal segment to urine results in a number of metabolic changes depending on the type of bowel used. Changes are more pronounced in continent reservoirs, where urine is in contact with the intestinal mucosa (with associated ion exchange) for prolonged periods of time. Use of the non-terminal ileum, which is most common, results in a hyperchloraemic metabolic acidosis that is subclinical 90% of the time. Malabsorption due to intestinal segment removal can cause vitamin deficiency (particularly vitamin B12) from five years after reconstruction. The impact of these metabolic changes on pregnancy is unclear.

The theoretical risk of the gravid uterus stretching or compressing the mesentery of an intestinal flap to the point of compromising the blood supply of that flap has not been borne out in clinical practice. As the gravid uterus enlarges, the pedicles of reconstructions based in the right iliac fossa (RIF), particularly ileal conduits and RIF catheterisable conduits are displaced laterally. The pedicles of reconstructions based towards the midline (for example, augmentation cystoplasties and neobladders) elongate over the gravid uterus and care must be taken not to injure these during CS [19].

As a rule, reconstruction of the urinary tract is not inherently a contraindication to vaginal delivery (although in reconstructed bladder neck cases specifically, elective CS must be considered more strongly due to recurrence of UI if damaged during vaginal delivery). When CS is planned, for the majority of cases a standard lower segment CS remains appropriate, switching to an upper segment CS early if access is compromised by adhesions or the reconstruction. In select cases (such as rectus sheath tunnelled Mitrofanoff), a supraumbilical midline incision with planned upper segment CS is the most appropriate option. A urologist should be requested to attend to assist in women who have had a previous abdominal reconstructive procedure [19].

Upper urinary tract complications are more common in urinary tract reconstructions, particularly urinary tract infections (UTIs), but management of these is the same as in the general obstetric population.

7.4 Renal Transplant

7.4.1 Effects of Transplant on Pregnancy

Pregnancy in a renal transplant patient has a 71–76% live birth rate [20–22], and with incidence of conception ranging from 0.9–7% in dialysis dependent end-stage renal failure patients, transplantation remains the best contributor to fertility in end-stage renal failure patients, restoring the disrupted hypothalamic-gonadal axis in as little as six months. The pre-conception optimisation of fertility and of graft survival in the renal transplant patient is beyond the scope of this chapter, and not addressed.

Optimised renal transplant patients remain at risk of complications common to all pregnancies, as well as those specific to the presence of the graft (Table 7.3). However, the latter, though less familiar to the obstetrician, are typically of little clinical significance in the well managed patient, while the former remain at profoundly increased risks.

Table 7.3 Risks of renal transplant in pregnancy

Maternal		Fetal	
Usual complications at increased risk	Transplant specific	Usual complications at increased risk [14]	Transplant specific
Pre-eclampsia	Allograft function deterioration	Premature delivery (13-fold)	Immunosuppressive medication side effects
Hypertension		Low birth weight (12-fold)	
		Decreased size for gestational age (5-fold)	

Statistically significant, but not clinically significant in isolation, the change in graft function from pre-conception to post-pregnancy is minimal, with a mean increase in serum creatinine of 12.4 µmols/l only. More important are the six-fold increased risk of pre-eclampsia [23], and the increased risk of development of hypertension with sequelae of increased risk both to the mother (graft loss) and fetus (intra-uterine growth retardation and preterm delivery) [24]. Low dose aspirin reduces the risk of pre-eclampsia and should be initiated in all renal transplant patients; for those with a blood pressure persistently higher than 140/90 mmHg, antihypertensives should be initiated, avoiding angiotensin converting enzyme inhibitors due to the risk of subsequent oligohydramnios and pulmonary hypoplasia.

The expected proteinuria in pregnancy is significantly higher in renal transplant patients, particularly in the third trimester, when it can commonly be greater than 500 mg/24 hours [25]. This, alongside calcineurin inhibitors causing hyperuricaemia at baseline, and acute graft rejection being an alternative diagnosis for abrupt worsening of both proteinuria and hypertension all make recognition of pre-eclampsia in the renal transplant patient a diagnostic dilemma. It is never safe to attribute these findings solely to the presence of the renal transplant; thus, these factors likely contribute both to the reported increased rate of pre-eclampsia, and to the increased rate of CS and preterm delivery discussed below.

Ultimately, the management of the pregnant renal transplant patient is complex and should take place within the multidisciplinary team setting, including obstetricians, transplant nephrologists and neonatologists.

7.4.2 Labour and Delivery

Vaginal delivery is preferred over CS, with the indications for CS the same as any other obstetric case. However, the rate of CS in renal transplant recipients is certainly higher than the general population: worldwide, almost thrice at 62.6% [20](vs 21.1% [26]), and 64% (vs 24%) in the United Kingdom population specifically [22]. These figures go hand-in-hand with an increased rate of preterm (<37 weeks) delivery at 52% (6.5x increased risk), and a 24% small for gestational age rate, as well as the higher rate of pre-eclampsia discussed previously. The presence of a renal transplant as the sole indication for CS has been reported but should be avoided.

The position of the (single) transplanted renal unit is typically on the right side of the greater pelvis, retroperitoneally, with extra peritoneal passage of the ureter to the dome of the bladder. It does not therefore contribute to obstruction of labour. Although best practice would involve peripartum involvement of transplant surgeons, with or without imaging to delineate transplant anatomy, reports of injuries to renal transplants during CS are uncommon – some authors advocate a midline incision to further reduce the risk of injury, but the majority consider Pfannenstiel incisions safe [27].

7.4.3 Immunosuppressive Agents During the Perinatal Period

Immunosuppression of the pregnant renal transplant recipient patient requires close involvement of a transplant nephrologist with an interest in obstetrics as all immunosuppressive agents cross into the fetal circulation [28]. Regarding breastfeeding, azathioprine, cyclosporine, prednisone and tacrolimus are all considered safe [29]. Belatacep, mycophenolic acid, everolimus and sirolimus should be avoided due to a lack of evidence rather than evidence of harm.

7.5 Congenital Anomalies of the Urinary Tract

Numerous congenital anomalies of the urinary tract can subsequently impact on pregnancy, with these impacts either related to the conditions themselves or to associated reconstruction of the urinary tract using bowel (with the implications of this outlined previously). Patients born with exstrophy-epispadias complex, cloaca, spinal dysraphism, sacral agenesis, cerebral palsy, imperforate anus and congenital vesicoureteric reflux (VUR) (with or without small capacity bladders and UI), subsequently achieving pregnancy have all been reported [30, 31]. As a rule, after reconstruction of the lower urinary tract for congenital abnormalities, vaginal delivery is not associated with significantly increased risk, and should be considered before CS.

7.5.1 Exstrophy-Epispadias Complex

This is a spectrum of disorders ranging from the rare (approximately 1 in 450 000–500 000 in females), but less clinically severe complete epispadias; to the less common, clinically intermediate form, bladder exstrophy (approximately 1 in 120000–150000 in females); to the most extreme form, cloacal exstrophy (approximately 1 in 200000–400000 genetic females).

Attributable to the relative rarity of the exstrophy-epispadias complex in females, literature on this cohort tends to be limited to a small number of case series only [30, 32, 33]. Despite this, some conclusions can be drawn:

1. Though conception rates are lower than the general population, successful conception has been reported, with lifetime rates of 66–77% [32, 33]
2. There is a higher rate of breech presentations compared to the general population (57% vs 4%) [32]
3. There is probably a higher first trimester miscarriage rate (29% vs 21%)
4. Delayed/difficult conception is also seen in 29% (attributable to associated paramesonephric duct defects)
5. There is a significantly higher risk of procidentia (up to 50% in some series) [33]
6. Where there are no indications for CS, vaginal delivery is a safe, valid option

7.5.2 Persistent Cloaca

A more common condition and unrelated to cloacal exstrophy despite the similar name, persistent cloaca occurs only in females (1 in 20 000–25 000). Despite congenital failure of the embryonic cloaca to subsequently divide from a single common channel into the urinary, genital and intestinal tracts, pregnancies have been reported after reconstruction, albeit too few to draw meaningful conclusions from [31]. These cases, being so rare, will certainly require urological input peripartum, with CS the recommended method of delivery.

7.5.3 Spinal Dysraphism

The obstetric implications of failure of the lower spine to close and any associated neurogenic bladder are two-fold – firstly, the impact of any previous augmentation of the neurogenic bladder (for example a Mitrofanoff or augmentation cystoplasty) as outlined in the *Urinary Diversions and Mitrofanoffs During Pregnancy* section above, and secondly the impact of the dysraphism on pain management, particularly the inability to have an epidural [30]. For these reasons, an elective general anaesthetic CS may be considered, as the usual methods of pain control during labour will not be viable, and planned availability of urological input will need to be considered.

7.5.4 Congenital Vesicoureteric Reflux (CVUR)

The impact of CVUR reflux on pregnancy is variable and similarly, the need for intervention for CVUR is dependent on the disease phenotype. All are more likely to experience UTIs during pregnancy, regardless of any previous surgical intervention. The three main risk factors for poorer fetal outcomes are evidence of renal scarring, hypertension and markedly poor pre-existing renal function, with renal scarring associated with gestational hypertension (up to 42%), pre-eclampsia (up to 33%) and birth weights of <2500 g (up to 20%) [34, 35]. Regarding baseline renal function, some advocate counselling towards early pregnancy in patients with a rising creatinine before it reaches the apparent tipping point of 200 µmol/l (particularly if hypertensive), above which there is an increased risk of fetal growth retardation or intra-uterine death, as well as more frequent marked deterioration in renal function and new onset hypertension, with this cohort ultimately much more likely to develop end-stage renal disease [35]. Other than close observation of renal function, obstetric management is not expected to differ from the general population.

7.6 Conclusion

A variety of urogynaecological and urological problems can impact pregnancy and delivery. Multidisciplinary involvement is key to optimising outcome.

Clinical Governance Issues

- Women with a first degree relative with pelvic floor dysfunction should be offered PFMT from 20 weeks of pregnancy
- Offer delivery by CS to women who have had a previous surgical procedure for SUI
- Indwelling catheterisation is recommended for 12 hours after regional anaesthetic for delivery or perineal repair
- Consider urinary retention as a cause of severe pain post-partum
- Pregnancy after renal transplantation is associated with higher maternal, fetal and neonatal morbidity and these pregnancies require multidisciplinary input
- Multidisciplinary working with urology is important for safe Caesarean delivery in women with a history of surgery for urinary tract reconstruction or congenital urinary tract anomalies

---

References

1   A. Rajavuori, J. P. Repo, A. Häkkinen, et al. Maternal risk factors of urinary incontinence during pregnancy and postpartum: A prospective cohort study. *European Journal of Obstetrics &*
Gynecology and Reproductive Biology, **8** (2021), 100138. PMC8605044.

2   K. L. Lin, C. J. Shen, M. P. Wu, et al. Comparison of low urinary tract symptoms during pregnancy between primiparous and multiparous women.

BioMed Research International, (2014), 303697.

3   K. Patel, J. B. Long, S. S. Boyd and K. H. Kjerulff. Natural history of urinary incontinence from first childbirth to 30-months postpartum. *Archives of Gynecology and Obstetrics,* **30** (2021), 713–24.

4   L. E. Giugale, P. A. Moalli, T. P. Canavan, L. A. Meyn and S. S. Oliphant. Prevalence and predictors of urinary incontinence at 1 year postpartum. *Female Pelvic Medicine and Reconstructive Surgery,* **27** (2021), e436–e441.

5   B. T. Haylen, D. Ridder de, R. M. Freeman, et al. An International Urogynecological Association (IUGA)/ International Continence Society (ICS) joint report on the terminology for female pelvic floor dysfunction. *Neurourology and Urodynamics,* **29** (2010), 4–20.

6   S. J. Woodley, P. Lawrenson, R. Boyle, et al. Pelvic floor muscle training for preventing and treating urinary and faecal incontinence in antenatal and postnatal women. *Cochrane Database of Systematic Reviews,* (2020), Art. No.: CD007471.

7   National Institute for Health and Care Excellence. *NICE Guideline NG210: Pelvic Floor Dysfunction: Prevention and Non-Surgical Management.* (2021). www.nice.org.uk/guidance/ng210/resources/pelvic-floor-dysfunction-prevention-and-nonsurgical-management-pdf-66143768482501

8   A. Pradhan, D. G. Tincello and R. Kearney. Childbirth after pelvic floor surgery: Analysis of Hospital Episode Statistics in England, 2002–2008. *British Journal of Obstetrics and Gynaecology,* **120** (2013), 200–4.

9   S. A. Tulokas, P. Rahkola-Soisalo, M. Gissler, T. S. Mikkola and M. J. Mentula. Pregnancy and delivery after mid-urethral sling operation. *International Urogynecology Journal,* **32** (2021), 179–86.

10   J. P. Shah and P. Dasgupta. Voiding difficulties and retention. In S. L. Stanton and A. K. Monga eds., *Clinical Urogynaecology.*

(London: Churchill Livingstone, 2000), pp. 259–72.

11   J. N. Panicker, R. Anding, S. Arlandis, et al. Do we understand voiding dysfunction in women? Current understanding and future perspectives: ICI-RS 2017. *Neurourology and Urodynamics,* **37** (2018), S75–S85.

12   S. Yip, D. Sahota, M. Pang, et al. Postpartum urinary retention. *Acta Obstetricia et Gynecologica Scandinavica,* **83** (2004), 881–91.

13   A. Rantell, N. Veit-Rubin, I. Giarenis, et al. Recommendations and future research initiative to optimize bladder management in pregnancy and childbirth International Consultation on Incontinence – Research society 2018. *Neurourology and Urodynamics,* **38** (2019), S104–S110.

14   Institute of Obstetricians and Gynaecologists (Royal College of Physicians of Ireland) and the Directorate of Clinical Strategy and Programmes (Health Service Executive of Ireland). *Clinical Practice Guideline: Urinary Retention: Management of Urinary Retention in Pregnancy, Post-Partum and After Gynaecological Surgery.* (2018). https://rcpi-live-cdn.s3.amazonaws.com/wp-content/uploads/2021/12/UR-guidelines-for-clinical-care-pathway-17.05.18.pdf

15   National Institute for Health and Care Excellence. *Clinical Guideline CG190: Intrapartum Care for Healthy Women and Babies.* (2017). www.nice.org.uk/guidance/cg190/resources/intrapartum-care-for-healthy-women-and-babies-pdf-35109866447557

16   National Institute for Health and Care Excellence. *NICE Guideline NG192: Caesarean Birth.* (2021). www.nice.org.uk/guidance/ng192/resources/caesarean-birth-pdf-66142078788805

17   P. Abrams, L. Cardozo, M. Fall, et al. The standardisation of terminology of lower urinary tract function: Report from the standardisation sub-committee of the International Continence Society.

Neurourology and Urodynamics, **21** (2002), 167–78.

18 S. M. Biers, C. Harding, M. Belal, et al. British Association of Urological Surgeons (BAUS) consensus document: Management of female voiding dysfunction. *BJU International,* **129** (2022), 151–9.

19 J. C. Thomas, A. N. Squiers and M. R. Kaufman. Sexual function and pregnancy in the female myelodysplasia patient. In H. M. Wood and D. Wood, eds., *Transition and Lifelong Care in Congenital Urology.* (Switzerland: Springer International Publishing, 2015), pp. 45–54.

20 S. Shah, R. L. Venkatesan, A. Gupta, et al. Pregnancy outcomes in women with kidney transplant: Metanalysis and systematic review. *BMC Nephrology,* **20** (2019), 24.

21 L. A. Coscia, S. Constantinescu, M. J. Moritz, et al. Report from the National Transplantation Pregnancy Registry (NTPR): Outcomes of pregnancy after transplantation. *Clinical Transplantation,* (2010), 65–85.

22 K. Bramham, C. Nelson-Piercy, H. Gao, et al. Pregnancy in renal transplant recipients: A UK national cohort study. *Clinical Journal of the American Society of Nephrology,* **8** (2013), 290–8.

23 S. Shah and P. Verma. Overview of pregnancy in renal transplant patients. *International Journal of Nephrology,* (2016), 4539342.

24 N. Sibanda, J. D. Briggs, J. M. Davison, et al. Pregnancy after organ transplantation: A report from the UK transplant pregnancy registry. *Transplantation,* **83** (2007), 1301–7.

25 J. M. Davison. The effect of pregnancy on kidney function in renal allograft recipients. *Kidney International,* **27** (1985), 74–9.

26 A. P. Betran, J. Ye, A-B. Moller, et al. Trends and projections of Caesarean section rates: Global and regional estimates. *BMJ Global Health,* **6** (2021), e005671.

27 C. E. Gordon and V. Tatsis. Shearing-force injury of a kidney transplant graft during Cesarean section: A case report and review of the literature. *BMC Nephrology,* **20** (2019), 94.

28 L. A. Coscia, S. Constantinescu, J. M. Davison, et al. Immunosuppressive drugs and fetal outcome. *Best Practice Research: Clinical Obstetrics & Gynaecology,* **28** (2014), 1174–87.

29 S. Constantinescu, A. Pai, L. A. Coscia, et al. Breast-feeding after transplantation. *Best Practice Research: Clinical Obstetrics & Gynaecology,* **28** (2014), 1163–73.

30 T. J. Greenwell, S. N. Venn, S. Creighton, et al. Pregnancy after lower urinary tract reconstruction for congenital abnormalities. *BJU International,* **92** (2003), 773–7.

31 R. J. Rintala. Congenital cloaca: Long-term follow-up results with emphasis on outcomes beyond childhood. *Seminars in Pediatric Surgery,* **25** (2016), 112–16.

32 R. Deans, F. Banks, L-M. Liao, et al. Reproductive outcomes in women with classic bladder exstrophy: An observational cross-sectional study. *American Journal of Obstetrics and Gynecology,* **206** (2012), e1–6.

33 A. M. Giron, C. C. Passerotti, H. Nguyen, et al. Bladder exstrophy: Reconstructed female patients achieving normal pregnancy and delivering normal babies. *International Brazilian Journal of Urology,* **37** (2011), 605–10.

34 P. Jungers. Reflux nephropathy and pregnancy. *Baillière's Clinical Obstetrics and Gynaecology,* **8** (1994), 425–42.

35 J. G. Hollowell. Outcome of pregnancy in women with a history of vesico-ureteric reflux. *BJU International,* **102** (2008), 780–4.

Chapter

8

Previous Third and Fourth Degree Tears

Nicola Adanna Okeahialam, Abdul H. Sultan,
Ranee Thakar

8.1 Background

Obstetric anal sphincter injuries (OASIs), which is the collective term for third or fourth degree tears, are vaginal birth-related perineal injuries that are classified anatomically based on the extent of injury to the external anal sphincter (EAS), internal anal sphincter (IAS) and anal mucosa (Table 8.1) [1]. A national survey of 215 maternity units in the UK by Thiagamoorthy et al. [2] found the incidence of OASI to be 2.9%, with this rate being significantly higher in primiparous women compared to multiparous (6.1% vs 1.7%). Furthermore, population-based studies in the UK, Australia, Denmark, Norway, Sweden and Finland have shown that the recorded rates of OASIs have increased [3–5]. While this increase is likely to be due to improved clinical detection and reporting of OASI, the contribution of recent changes in practice of the management of the second stage of labour needs to be explored [6].

Risk factors for OASI include Asian, Indian and Filipino ethnicity, short maternal stature, an increased second stage of labour, assisted vaginal birth, midline episiotomy, occipito-posterior fetal head position, increased fetal birth weight and previous OASI [7]. A recent systematic review by Barba et al. [8] found that across 15 observational studies (697 082 women), the average rate of recurrent OASI (rOASI) was 5.0% with a range of 1.0–10.7%. Significant risk factors identified included maternal age, gestational age, occiput posterior presentation, oxytocin augmentation, assisted delivery and shoulder dystocia.

It is well documented that OASIs are associated with both short- and long-term anal incontinence. Bols et al. [9] performed a systematic review on risk factors associated with anal incontinence, with a follow-up period ranging from three months to ten years and found that OASI was strongly associated with anal incontinence in the post-natal period. The aetiology of anal incontinence is multifactorial, and may also be due to several factors including irritable bowel symptoms and neuropathy [10]. Anal sphincter integrity is also an important factor in maintaining continence. Primary anal sphincter repair at delivery can often be inadequate, characterised as a persistent defect on ultrasound in approximately 60% of cases, with 40% of women reporting anal incontinence [11]. Medical comorbidities such as inflammatory bowel disease can also affect the anorectum causing anal incontinence [12]. Although ulcerative colitis typically extends from the anorectum, up to 80% of patients with Crohn's disease will have perianal involvement [13]. Therefore, maintenance of anal sphincter and pelvic floor function in these patients with anorectal disease is imperative. To conserve anal sphincter function, maintain quality of life and the impact on future mode of delivery, obstetricians should be familiar with any pathology that affects the anal sphincter complex, including OASIs.

Table 8.1 Perineal trauma classification recommended by the Royal College of Obstetricians and Gynaecologists

Degree	Injury
Intact	No visible tear
First	Perineal skin only
Second	Perineal muscles but not involving the anal sphincter
Third	Anal sphincter complex 3a – less than 50% of the EAS thickness torn 3b – more than 50% of the EAS thickness torn 3c – both EAS and IAS torn
Fourth	Anal sphincter complex and anal mucosa

In this chapter, we will assess the current evidence base for the management of women with previous OASIs in the antenatal, intrapartum and post-partum period, the complications associated with OASIs and recommendations for subsequent delivery.

8.1.1 Antenatal

The management of subsequent pregnancies in women with previous OASIs is an important consideration for both the clinician and the woman. This is due to concerns surrounding the onset or potential deterioration of anorectal symptoms and recurrence of OASI. At present, there are ten published national guidelines regarding the management and prevention of OASI from the UK, USA, Australia, Austria, Canada, Denmark, Germany and Ireland, which provide advice concerning future pregnancies and mode of delivery, albeit conflicting [14]. Counselling surrounding the subsequent mode of delivery (vaginal or elective caesarean birth) should be individualised, taking into account tear grade, the severity of anorectal incontinence and the woman's wishes in an informed manner [15].

Women with previous OASIs may experience symptoms including involuntary loss of faeces (faecal incontinence), involuntary loss of gas (flatus incontinence) and a sudden desire to defaecate that is difficult to defer (faecal urgency) [16]. A prospective study by Gommeson et al. [17] found that in a cohort of 189 women, reviewed 12 months post-partum, those with a higher grade of OASI were at increased risk of experiencing anal incontinence. Overall, 13.6% (n = 12) of those with a 3a tear developed symptoms and 15.2% (n = 10), 35.0% (n = 7) and 33.3% (n = 5) of women with 3b, 3c and fourth degree tears, respectively, developed symptoms. Furthermore, the risk of anal incontinence was over four-fold higher in women sustaining 3c and fourth degree tears [17]. This is probably secondary to involvement of the IAS, injury to which has been shown to be predictive of faecal incontinence. Mahoney et al. [18] found that 9% of women with injury to the IAS had severe incontinence symptoms, compared with only 1.4% of those with no IAS defect. Management of anal incontinence symptoms secondary to OASI in the antenatal period is always conservative in the form of pelvic muscle floor training (PFMT). However, the evidence to support antenatal PFMT is limited with a Cochrane review by Woodley et al. [19] demonstrating that it does not improve anal incontinence symptoms in late pregnancy. However, this review included women of any parity and did not perform subgroup analysis based on a history of OASIs [19].

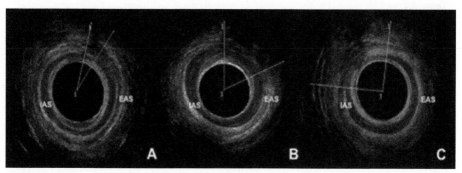

Fig 8.1 (A) Endoanal ultrasound showing a scar within the external anal sphincter (EAS) measuring 20°(≤1 hour (h)). (B) Endoanal ultrasound showing an EAS defect measuring 63°, (~2 hours). (C) Endoanal ultrasound showing an internal (IAS) and EAS measuring 96°, (>3h in size). Reproduced with permission from Okeahialam et al. [24]

Anal incontinence also affects 24% of people with inflammatory bowel disease [20]. Norton et al. [20] reported, in their population-based study of 10 000 patients registered with the *Crohn's & Colitis UK* charity, that the risk of anal incontinence was significantly increased by 30% in women. Furthermore, the risk of anal incontinence in women was increased by approximately 50% in those who had experienced at least one vaginal birth and this can persist at least five years after birth, irrespective of Crohn's typology [20, 21]. International guidelines recommend that there is no contraindication to vaginal delivery, except for women with active perianal disease or active rectal involvement, where caesarean birth is recommended. An ileoanal pouch or an ileorectal anastomosis is a relative indication for a caesarean birth [22]. Active perineal disease has been shown to increase the risk of severe perineal laceration [23]. A retrospective study by Hatch et al. [23] of 6 797 669 births between 1998–2009 showed that of 2 882 (0.04%) women who had Crohn's disease, the risk of fourth degree tear was higher in those with perianal disease.

Endoanal ultrasound (EAUS) is considered the gold standard investigation for the evaluation of the anal sphincter complex and residual effects following repair of OASI [16]. Images obtained from women with anal sphincter defects at three-months post-partum are shown in Figure 8.1.

Anal manometry can be performed to assess anal sphincter function [10]. Anal sphincter dysfunction and subsequent symptoms can also be secondary to pudendal neuropathy or a combination of sphincter injury and neuropathy [25]. The pudendal nerve, which innervates the EAS, can be stretched and/or compressed by the fetal head during labour, a prolonged second stage or assisted vaginal birth throughout the nerve's course, including its perineal terminal branch [26]. This neuropathy is usually temporary and resolves spontaneously in the majority of women within six months [27]. We evaluated EAUS, anal manometry and anorectal symptoms in 146 women three months following OASIs and also in the antenatal period of a subsequent pregnancy (average of 30 months between the two assessment points). There was no change in anal sphincter defect size over time. Moreover, anal manometry pressures and anorectal symptoms improved. This improvement was significant in women with no residual sphincter defect on ultrasound [24]. This highlights that after OASI, anorectal symptoms improve with time, even in the context of pregnancy, which has no detrimental effect on anal sphincter

Table 8.2 Published protocols in the UK regarding mode of delivery recommendations following OASI

Unit	Criteria for elective Caesarean birth recommendation
Croydon University Hospital, London [29]	Asymptomatic or mild anal incontinence symptoms with EAS defect and low incremental rise on anal manometry from resting to squeeze (<20 mmHg)
St Mary's Hospital, London [30]	Anal incontinence symptoms or anal sphincter defect (IAS or EAS) or low resting pressure on anal manometry (<40 mmHg) or low incremental rise from resting to squeeze (<20 mmHg)
Norfolk and Norwich [31]	Asymptomatic with EAS defect and low incremental rise on anal manometry from resting to squeeze <20 mmHg If symptomatic, only one abnormal investigation is required (EAS defect or incremental rise)
Dublin, Ireland [32]	Severe symptoms (Wexner score >5) and ultrasound defects greater than one quadrant For women with ultrasound defects less than 1 quadrant but symptomatic or women who had ultrasound defects >1 quadrant on ultrasound but were asymptomatic, anal sphincter tone on digital rectal examination, anal manometry and patient wishes are taken into consideration

integrity. Specialist investigations such as EAUS and anal manometry are not readily available in all obstetric units. Therefore, in centres where they are not available, antenatal counselling regarding mode of delivery should be based on anal incontinence symptom severity taking into account tear grade; particularly fourth degree tears [15, 28]. Several specialist units have published their protocols with mode of delivery recommendations [28]. Table 8.2 outlines published protocols from four units in the UK and Figure 8.2 illustrates a protocol from one of these units [29]. It is imperative that women are informed about the risk of rOASI in the antenatal period and they should be informed that this risk is higher with assisted vaginal birth, previous fourth degree tears and a fetal birth weight over 4 kg [33].

Recurrent OASI is not without consequence, as it is associated with worsening of anal sphincter function demonstrated using anal manometry and anal sphincter integrity on EAUS [34]. However, at short-term (12 weeks) and long-term follow-up (10 years), studies have found that rOASI is not associated with a significant difference in anal incontinence prevalence or severity [34, 35].

In cases of rectal buttonhole tears, although by definition, they are not OASIs per se, antenatal counselling should be provided in a subsequent pregnancy with regards to the mode of delivery [36]. A rectal buttonhole tear is an isolated tear of the anal epithelium or rectal mucosa and vagina without involving the anal sphincter [37]. However, on rare occasions these can occur concurrently with OASIs [36]. In women with concurrent anal sphincter trauma, management in a subsequent pregnancy should follow published protocols regarding the management of OASI [28, 36]. Due to a paucity of evidence, in cases of isolated rectal buttonhole tears, women should be counselled surrounding the risks and benefits of a caesarean in comparison to vaginal birth so an informed decision regarding their desired mode of delivery can be made [36].

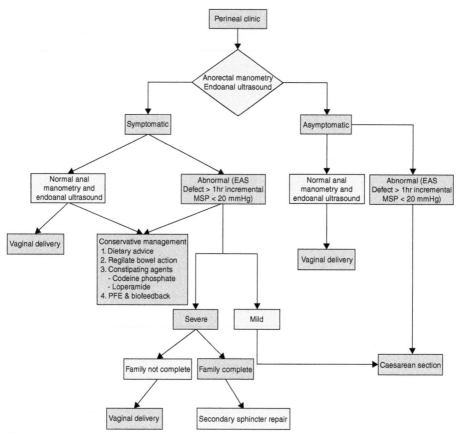

Fig 8.2 Protocol used to aid the recommended mode of delivery decision in a subsequent pregnancy following OASI. Reproduced with permission from Jordan et al. [29]

Another potential but rare sequelae of previous OASI and rectal buttonhole tears is the formation of an anogenital fistula [36, 37]. Obstetric fistulae usually occur either immediately following vaginal delivery and perineal repair with an unrecognised recto-vaginal fistula, or 1–2 weeks following delivery, as a result of wound infection, subsequent inflammation and wound breakdown of a fourth degree tear. Not all fistulae will require surgical intervention as 50% of all small fistulae will heal spontaneously [38]. However, in a subsequent pregnancy following fistula surgery, caesarean birth is generally recommended [39].

8.1.2 Intrapartum

Although the majority of women with previous OASIs will deliver with no concerns, the risk of rOASI in a subsequent vaginal birth can be reduced with modification of obstetric practice. There is no agreed international consensus about interventions that can be applied intrapartum to reduce the risk of rOASI. However, there is evidence from countries such as the UK, Norway and Denmark that a reduction in the rate of OASI can be achieved through quality improvement initiatives involving the training of clinicians in manual perineal protection and mediolateral episiotomy [40–42]. For example, in 2018, the Royal College of Obstetricians and Gynaecologists (RCOG) and the Royal College of Midwives (RCM) supported the implementation and evaluation of the OASI Care Bundle in 16 maternity units across the UK. The OASI Care Bundle consisted of four components, including antenatal education, manual perineal protection, mediolateral episiotomy if clinically indicated and systemic per vaginal and rectal examination to assess for anal sphincter injury. The implementation of this initiative significantly reduced the risk of OASI by 20% [42].

Manual perineal protection (MPP) can be used to control the birth of the fetal head and to reduce its presenting diameter, thereby controlling the stretch on the perineum. However, a meta-analysis by Bulchandani et al. (40) found inconsistent results between existing randomised control trials (RCTs) (n = 3) and non-RCTs (n = 3) investigating the effect of MPP on the risk of OASI. Although the pooled incidence of OASI was 37% and 55% lower with MPP in the RCTs and non-RCTs, respectively, this protective effect was only significant in the non-RCTs. It is important to note that with the RCTs, no study was designed with the primary aim of assessing the effect of MPP on OASI. Furthermore, clinician compliance could not be controlled for and the MPP technique with regards to initiation time and perineal support at the time of shoulder delivery differed across the studies [43]. The use of prophylactic mediolateral episiotomy (MLE) in the prevention of rOASI is also unclear. The previous meta-analysis was unable to analyse the pooled effect of episiotomy as the included studies did not provide sufficient data surrounding episiotomy type (midline, mediolateral or lateral) [33]. However, the retrospective cohort study of 209 584 singletons, term, cephalic vaginal births, subsequently published by D'Souza et al. [44] suggested the use of MLE was protective against rOASI and reduced the risk of re-injury by 80%. Moreover, the authors reported that overall, eight MLE's were required to prevent one additional rOASI in any birth type (spontaneous and assisted vaginal birth). In addition, in spontaneous vaginal births alone, ten MLE's were required to prevent one additional rOASI. In women with inflammatory bowel disease and active perianal disease undergoing vaginal delivery, there is evidence that episiotomy also reduces the risk of OASI [23]. However, episiotomy may actually trigger perianal disease in those with no pre-existing perianal disease 1–2 months following vaginal delivery [45]. Therefore, taking into account additional associated risks with routine episiotomy including blood loss, perineal pain and dyspareunia, the need for mediolateral episiotomy should be assessed at the time of delivery if severe perineal laceration is anticipated, considering the preferences of the woman [46].

8.1.3 Post-Partum

Pelvic floor muscle training in the post-partum is often routinely advised for women with OASIs. Interestingly, the effect of post-natal pelvic floor muscle training on anal incontinence was uncertain in the meta-analysis performed by Woodley et al. [19]. However, this population included all women with anal incontinence and not those specifically with a history of OASI. Results of the efficacy of post-partum pelvic floor muscle training in women with OASI, commenced two weeks after index delivery are positive, as pelvic floor muscle training was shown to significantly improve anal incontinence symptoms from 2–12 weeks [47]. However, the impact of pelvic floor muscle training in the long term or in women with previous OASIs following a subsequent delivery is yet to be evaluated. As pelvic floor muscle training is not harmful and compliance is important for its effectiveness, women with a history of OASI should be encouraged to do pelvic floor and anal muscle exercises.

In women experiencing significant anal incontinence, if conservative measures have failed, surgical measures should be considered. However, this is dependent on whether the woman has completed her family or not. Secondary anal sphincter repair is an option in cases of residual structural defects in the anal sphincter following OASI. Barbosa et al. [48] suggested that by 18-year follow-up, a large proportion of women experienced a deterioration of symptoms and reported significant anal incontinence and reduced quality of life. From their cohort of 255 women, flatus and faecal incontinence were reported by 97% and 75%, respectively. Other management options include sacral neuromodulation. Rydningen et al. [49] found that in women with previous OASI, anal incontinence and concurrent urinary incontinence, sacral neuromodulation was effective in improving symptoms and symptom-related quality of life at 12 months. However, access to these options usually requires referral to a tertiary centre.

8.2 Clinical Dilemmas

Anal incontinence can have a significant physical and emotional impact on women. Planned Caesarean section in a subsequent delivery for all women with a history OASI may be a method to prevent future anal incontinence. However, there is no clear agreed consensus. The EPIC study, a population-based study of urinary incontinence, overactive bladder and other lower urinary tract symptoms in five countries, indicated that planned caesarean birth in comparison to a vaginal birth in a subsequent delivery did not significantly impact the incidence of anal incontinence at eight months post-partum [50]. However, as follow-up was short, anal incontinence incidence at long-term follow-up was not addressed, particularly considering the effect of the menopause on the pelvic floor. More research is required into the preventative strategies against anal incontinence in women with a history of OASI. However, a RCT to address long-term outcomes, with a large enough sample size would prove difficult. Additionally, women may have a varying extent of damage to the components of the anal sphincter and the symptoms vary based on many factors such as concomitant neuropathy and underlying disorders such as irritable bowel syndrome. In the presence of limited evidence, when counselling women in a subsequent delivery, they must also be fully informed about the pros and cons of the mode of birth.

8.3 Conclusion

The consequences of OASI can lead to long-term physical and psychological sequelae. Although uncommon, rOASI may increase the risk of future anal incontinence due to its negative effect on anal sphincter integrity and function. Therefore, obstetricians should be well versed in counselling women in a subsequent pregnancy and be aware of factors that may increase the risk of further anal sphincter disruption, so that obstetric practice can be modified.

The recommended mode of delivery in asymptomatic women in a subsequent pregnancy is usually vaginal, while in women, with significant anorectal symptoms, caesarean section is generally recommended. However, in tertiary units where specialist investigations are available, this decision may also consider anal sphincter integrity and function using modalities such as EAUS and anorectal physiology. caesarean birth in a subsequent pregnancy may be a preventative strategy against the development of anal incontinence in the short term, however, the development of symptoms in the long term is yet to be evaluated. Therefore, the cumulative risks of caesarean and repeat caesarean birth in future pregnancies need to be discussed during counselling.

Clinical Governance Issues

- Women should be made aware that the risk of repeat OASI is approximately 5%
- Women who opt for a vaginal birth should be informed about risk factors for OASI and repeat OASI such as increased maternal age, assisted vaginal birth and increased birthweight
- Health-care professionals should be aware of the pros and cons of vaginal and caesarean birth and should discuss these with women to allow them to make an informed decision
- Clinicians should be aware of intrapartum factors which increase the risk of OASI, so that obstetric practice can be modified
- Women should be encouraged to do pelvic floor muscle training and continue it in the long term
- When women require surgery for anal incontinence, this should be performed when her family is complete. In cases where women are unsure if their family is complete, they should be advised a caesarean section may be required

References

1   A. H. Sultan. Obstetric perineal injury and anal incontinence. *AVMA Medical & Legal Journal*, **5** (1999), 193–6.

2   G. Thiagamoorthy, A. Johnson, R. Thakar and A. H. Sultan. National survey of perineal trauma and its subsequent management in the United Kingdom. *International Urogynecology Journal*, **25** (2014), 1621–7.

3   K. Laine, M. Gissler and J. Pirhonen. Changing incidence of anal sphincter tears in four Nordic countries through the last decades. *European Journal of Obstetrics & Gynecology and Reproductive Biology*, **146** (2009), 71–5.

4   A. J. Ampt, J. B. Ford, C. L. Roberts and J. M. Morris. Trends in obstetric anal sphincter injuries and associated risk factors for vaginal singleton term births in New South Wales 2001–2009. *Australian and New Zealand Journal of Obstetrics and Gynaecology*, **53** (2013), 9–16.

5   I. Gurol-Urganci, D. Cromwell, L. Edozien, et al. Third- and fourth-degree perineal tears among primiparous women in England between 2000 and 2012: Time trends and risk factors. *BJOG: International Journal of Obstetrics & Gynaecology*, **120** (2013), 1516–25.

6   P. A. Baghurst. The case for retaining severe perineal tears as an indicator of the quality of obstetric care. *Australian and New Zealand Journal of Obstetrics and Gynaecology*, **53** (2013), 3–8.

7   T. C. Dudding, C. J. Vaizey and M. A. Kamm. Obstetric anal sphincter injury: Incidence, risk factors, and management. *Annals of Surgery*, **247** (2008), 224–37.

8   M. Barba, D. P. Bernasconi, S. Manodoro and M. Frigerio. Risk factors for obstetric anal sphincter injury recurrence: A systematic review and meta-analysis. *International Journal of Gynecology & Obstetrics*, **00** (2021), 1–8.

9 E. M. J. Bols, E. J. M. Hendriks, B. C. M. Berghmans, et al. A systematic review of etiological factors for postpartum fecal incontinence. *Acta Obstetricia et Gynecologica Scandinavica,* **89** (2010), 302–14.

10 S. M. Scott and P. J. Lunniss. Investigations of anorectal function. In A. H. Sultan, R. Thakar and D. E. Fenner, eds., *Perineal and Anal Sphincter Trauma: Diagnosis and Clinical Management* [Internet]. (New York; London: Springer, 2009), pp. 102–22. https://doi.org/10 .1007/978-1-84628-503-5

11 M. Sideris, T. McCaughey, J. G. Hanrahan, et al. Risk of obstetric anal sphincter injuries (OASIS) and anal incontinence: A meta-analysis. *European Journal of Obstetrics & Gynecology and Reproductive Biology,* **252** (2020), 303–12.

12 C. J. van der Woude, S. Kolacek, I. Dotan, et al. European evidenced-based consensus on reproduction in inflammatory bowel disease. *Journal of Crohn's and Colitis,* **4** (2010), 493–510.

13 B. Singh, N. J. McC Mortensen, D. P. Jewell and B. George. Perianal Crohn's disease. *British Journal of Surgery,* **91** (2004), 801–14.

14 J. C. Roper, N. Amber, O. Y. K. Wan, A. H. Sultan and R. Thakar. Review of available national guidelines for obstetric anal sphincter injury. *International Urogynecology Journal,* **31** (2020), 2247–59.

15 Royal College of Obstetrics and Gynaecology. *Management of Third and Fourth Degree Perineal Tears. Greentop Guideline Number 29* [Internet]. (RCOG Press, 2015). www.rcog.org.uk/globalassets/ documents/guidelines/gtg-29.pdf

16 A. H. Sultan, A. Monga, J. Lee, et al. An International Urogynecological Association (IUGA)/International Continence Society (ICS) joint report on the terminology for female anorectal dysfunction. *International Urogynecology Journal,* **28** (2017), 5–31.

17 D. Gommesen, EAa. Nohr, N. Qvist and Rasch V. Obstetric perineal ruptures – risk of anal incontinence among primiparous women 12 months postpartum: A prospective cohort study. *American Journal of Obstetrics and Gynecology,* **222** (2020), e1–e11.

18 R. Mahony, M. Behan, L. Daly, et al. Internal anal sphincter defect influences continence outcome following obstetric anal sphincter injury. *American Journal of Obstetrics and Gynecology,* **196** (2007), e1–e5.

19 S. Woodley, P. Lawrenson, R. Boyle, et al. Pelvic floor muscle training for preventing and treating urinary and faecal incontinence in antenatal and postnatal women. *Cochrane Database of Systematic Reviews* [Internet]. (John Wiley & Sons, Ltd., 2020). http://dx.doi.org/10.1002/ 14651858.CD007471.pub4

20 C. Norton, L. B. Dibley and P. Bassett. Faecal incontinence in inflammatory bowel disease: Associations and effect on quality of life. *Journal of Crohn's and Colitis,* **7** (2013), e302–11.

21 C. Mégier, C. Bourbao-Tournois, F. Perrotin, et al. Long-term evaluation of the impact of delivery modalities on anal continence in women with Crohn's disease. *Journal of Visceral Surgery* [Internet], (2021). www.sciencedirect.com/science/ article/pii/S1878788621001296

22 C. J. van der Woude, S. Ardizzone, M.B. Bengtson, et al. The second European evidenced-based consensus on reproduction and pregnancy in inflammatory bowel disease. *Journal of Crohn's and Colitis,* **9** (2015), 107–24.

23 Q. Hatch, B. J. Champagne, J. A. Maykel, et al. Crohn's Disease and pregnancy: The impact of perianal disease on delivery methods and complications. *Diseases of the Colon & Rectum,* **57** (2014), 174–8.

24 N. A. Okeahialam, R. Thakar and A. H. Sultan. Effect of a subsequent pregnancy on anal sphincter integrity and function after obstetric anal sphincter injury (OASI). *International Urogynecology Journal* [Internet], (2020). http://link .springer.com/10.1007/s00192-020- 04607-8

25 F. Lone, A. Sultan and R. Thakar. Obstetric pelvic floor and anal sphincter injuries. *Obstetrics & Gynecology*, **14** (2012), 257–66.

26 M. Jóźwik and M. Jóźwik. Partial denervation of the pelvic floor during term vaginal delivery. *International Urogynecology Journal*, **12** (2001), 81–2.

27 A. H. Sultan, M. A. Kamm and C. N. Hudson. Pudendal nerve damage during labour: Prospective study before and after childbirth. *BJOG: An International Journal of Obstetrics & Gynaecology*, **101** (1994), 22–8.

28 A. Taithongchai, R. Thakar and A. H. Sultan. Management of subsequent pregnancies following fourth-degree obstetric anal sphincter injuries (OASIS). *European Journal of Obstetrics & Gynecology and Reproductive Biology*, **250** (2020), 80–5.

29 P. A. Jordan, M. Naidu, R. Thakar and A. H. Sultan. Effect of subsequent vaginal delivery on bowel symptoms and anorectal function in women who sustained a previous obstetric anal sphincter injury. *International Urogynecology Journal*, **29** (2018), 1579–88.

30 R. Karmarkar, A. Bhide, A. Digesu, V. Khullar and R. Fernando. Mode of delivery after obstetric anal sphincter injury. *European Journal of Obstetrics & Gynecology and Reproductive Biology*, **194** (2015), 7–10.

31 C. Cassis, I. Giarenis, S. Mukhopadhyay and E. Morris. Mode of delivery following an OASIS and caesarean section rates. *European Journal of Obstetrics & Gynecology and Reproductive Biology*, **230** (2018), 28–31.

32 M. Fitzpatrick, M. Cassidy, M. L. Barassaud, et al. Does anal sphincter injury preclude subsequent vaginal delivery? *European Journal of Obstetrics & Gynecology and Reproductive Biology*, **198** (2016), 30–4.

33 S. Jha and V. Parker. Risk factors for recurrent obstetric anal sphincter injury (rOASI): A systematic review and meta-analysis. *International Urogynecology Journal*, **27** (2016), 849–57.

34 N. A. Okeahialam, R. Thakar, M. Naidu and A. H. Sultan. Outcome of anal symptoms and anorectal function following two obstetric anal sphincter injuries (OASIS) – a nested case-controlled study. *International Urogynecology Journal* [Internet], (2020). http://link.springer.com/10.1007/s00192-020-04377-3

35 R. A. Bøgeskov, C. N. A. Nickelsen and N. J. Secher. Anal incontinence in women with recurrent obstetric anal sphincter rupture: A case control study. *The Journal of Maternal-Fetal & Neonatal Medicine*, **28** (2015), 288–92.

36 J. C. Roper, R. Thakar and A. H. Sultan. Isolated rectal buttonhole tears in obstetrics: Case series and review of the literature. *International Urogynecology Journal* [Internet], (2020). http://link.springer.com/10.1007/s00192-020-04502-2

37 A. H. Sultan and C. Kettle. Diagnosis of perineal trauma. In A. H. Sultan, R. Thakar and D. E. Fenner, eds., *Perineal and Anal Sphincter Trauma*. (Springer, 2007), pp. 13–20.

38 R. Homsi, N. H. Daikoku, J. Littlejohn and C. R. Wheeless. Episiotomy: Risks of dehiscence and rectovaginal fistula. *Obstetrical & Gynecological Survey*, **49** (1994), 803–8.

39 A. H. Sultan and S. L. Stanton. Preserving the pelvic floor and perineum during childbirth-elective caesarean section? *BJOG: An International Journal of Obstetrics & Gynaecology*, **103** (1996), 731–4.

40 E. Hals, P. Øian, T. Pirhonen, et al. A multicenter interventional program to reduce the incidence of anal sphincter tears. *Obstetrics & Gynecology*, **116** (2010), 901–8.

41 O. B. Rasmussen, A. Yding, Ø. J. Anh, C. Sander Andersen and J. Boris. Reducing the incidence of obstetric sphincter injuries using a hands-on technique: An interventional quality improvement

project. *BMJ Quality Improvement Reports,* **5** (2016), u217936.w7106.

42 L. Edozien, I. Gurol-Urganci, D. Cromwell, et al. Impact of third- and fourth-degree perineal tears at first birth on subsequent pregnancy outcomes: A cohort study. *BJOG: An International Journal of Obstetrics & Gynaecology,* **121** (2014), 1695–703.

43 S. Bulchandani, E. Watts, A. Sucharitha, D. Yates and K. Ismail. Manual perineal support at the time of childbirth: A systematic review and meta-analysis. *BJOG: International Journal of Obstetrics & Gynaecology,* **122** (2015), 1157–65.

44 J. C. D'Souza, A. Monga, D. G. Tincello, et al. Maternal outcomes in subsequent delivery after previous obstetric anal sphincter injury (OASI): A multi-centre retrospective cohort study. *International Urogynecology Journal* [Internet], (2019). http://link.springer.com/10.1007/s00192–019-03983-0

45 L. J. Brandt, S. G. Estabrook and J. F. Reinus. Results of a survey to evaluate whether vaginal delivery and episiotomy lead to perineal involvement in women with Crohn's disease. *American Journal of Gastroenterology,* **90** (1995), 1918–22.

46 G. Carroli and L. Mignini. Episiotomy for vaginal birth. In: *The Cochrane Collaboration,* ed., Cochrane Database of Systematic Reviews [Internet].

(Chichester, UK: John Wiley & Sons, Ltd., 2009), CD000081.pub2. https://doi.wiley.com/10.1002/14651858.CD000081.pub2

47 E. Von Bargen, M. J. Haviland, O. H. Chang, et al. Evaluation of postpartum pelvic floor physical therapy on obstetrical anal sphincter injury: A randomized controlled trial. *Female Pelvic Medicine and Reconstructive Surgery,* **27** (2021), 315–21.

48 M. Barbosa, M. Glavind-Kristensen, M. Moller Soerensen and P. Christensen. Secondary sphincter repair for anal incontinence following obstetric sphincter injury: Functional outcome and quality of life at 18 years of follow-up. *Colorectal Disease,* **22** (2020), 71–9.

49 M. B. Rydningen, S. Riise, T. Wilsgaard, R. O. Lindsetmo and S. Norderval. Sacral neuromodulation for combined faecal and urinary incontinence following obstetric anal sphincter injury. *Colorectal Disease,* **20** (2018), 59–67.

50 L. Abramowitz, L. Mandelbrot, A. Bourgeois Moine, et al. Cesarean section in the second delivery to prevent anal incontinence after asymptomatic obstetrical anal sphincter injury: The EPIC multicenter randomized trial. *BJOG: An International Journal of Obstetrics & Gynaecology,* (2020), 1471-0528.16452.

Chapter 9

Management of Post-Partum Retained Placental Remnants

Mary Connor, Priya Madhuvrata

9.1 Introduction

Inadvertent retention of products of conception (RPOC) occurs in 1–6% of all pregnancies, with 1% of post-partum women in high-income countries undergoing surgical treatment for suspected RPOC [1]. The precise definition of RPOC is problematic but can be taken as placental remnants persisting after initial removal or treatment following any pregnancy, and between 24 hours to 12 weeks after delivery. However, occasionally it may not be revealed for several months, partly because diagnosis can be difficult. It occurs more commonly following miscarriage or termination of pregnancy rather than vaginal delivery or Caesarean section (CS) [2]. It is estimated that with deliveries after 24 weeks' gestation approximately 3 800 to 15 200 of post-natal women in the UK (0.5–2% of all deliveries) are admitted to hospital each year with secondary post-partum haemorrhage (PPH). Half of these women (between 1 900 and 7 600) undergo surgical uterine evacuation of RPOC [1].

Histological confirmation of RPOC in women who undergo surgical treatment is relatively low, ranging from 37–80% depending upon the threshold used for surgical intervention [3, 4]. Surgical treatment can be hazardous with risks including uterine perforation, subsequent intra-uterine adhesion formation and even hysterectomy [3, 5, 6].

In the absence of randomised controlled trials (RCTs) there is insufficient high-quality evidence to form the basis of clear guidelines on the management of RPOC following any pregnancy at whatever gestation [1, 7]. Consequently, when considering the options for investigation and treatment, advice for management draws upon the published information that is available, including retrospective studies and the occasional systematic review. Most studies are not confined to a specific gestation and often combine results for treatment of RPOC following miscarriage, abortion or delivery.

9.2 Diagnosis

The presenting complaint with retained placental remnants is commonly secondary PPH, though symptoms may include lower abdominal pain and fever. The main differential diagnosis is with genital tract infection, but in this situation fever, tachycardia and abdominal pain predominate. Other causes to be considered when the blood loss is light are blood clots within the uterine cavity but also, though very rarely a problem, gestational trophoblastic disease (GTD) [8]. Most commonly, the blood loss with secondary PPH is not particularly heavy, though more than expected by the woman and her carers for the time since delivery and may be persistent and irregular. Occasionally, heavy vaginal bleeding is the presenting complaint and is clearly more serious and demands an immediate response. Besides RPOC, other causes of bleeding that should be considered include GTD and uterine vascular abnormalities such as subinvolution of the placental implantation site, pseudoaneurysm of the uterine artery and even arteriovenous malformations (AVM) (see Table 9.1) [8].

9.2.1 Ultrasonography

The first line investigation of secondary PPH is grey-scale ultrasonography where features of RPOC consist of variable amounts of echogenic or heterogeneous material within the endometrial cavity. An ultrasound scan (USS) can, at the very least, identify an empty uterine cavity, and the presence of an echogenic mass correlates with RPOC. This is especially so with an enlarged cavity diameter where the anteroposterior diameter is above the 90th centile, approximately 25 mm on days 1–7 post-partum [9].

Colour Doppler studies enable vascularity within the echogenic material to be assessed. Kamaya et al. [4] reported on a spectrum of vascularity with the probability of confirmed RPOC increasing with the degree of vascularity. However, the absence of vascularity within an echogenic mass does not exclude RPOCs; in this circumstance, it is difficult to differentiate RPOC from an intra-uterine blood clot. Monitoring of a thickened avascular endometrium by USS over a period of one to two weeks may help resolve this difficulty with a blood clot more likely to disappear spontaneously.

9.2.2 Other Diagnostic Investigations

MRI has a role when the USS results are inconclusive and symptoms fail to resolve with accurate assessment of vascularity [8]. In an emergency with very heavy vaginal bleeding, contrast-enhanced CT has a role and can help with diagnosis of uncommon conditions such as uterine pseudoaneurysm [8]. Diagnostic and interventional arteriography has a specific place for managing heavy active uterine bleeding and for extremely rare AVM [10].

Other rare conditions, such as GTD, can be suspected in the presence of a hypervascular uterine mass, and a very high serum β-human chorionic gonadotrophin (β-hCG) level makes this highly likely. Surgical treatment with removal of abnormal trophoblastic tissue enables histopathological confirmation of the diagnosis and initiation of appropriate treatment. A β-hCG level is not otherwise useful for determining the presence of RPOC postdelivery because it is likely to be negative, though occasionally a low level is obtained [11].

9.3 Causative Factors

Retained placenta tissue is generally attributed to one of the following pathophysiologies. A separated placenta may be trapped due to closure of the cervix prior to delivery of the placenta [12, 13]. Poor uterine contraction may prevent normal separation and contractile expulsion of the whole placenta [12–14]. Appropriate management with induction of adequate uterine contractions is generally followed by placental separation and its complete removal. In both these situations, provided that the placenta is removed intact rather than piecemeal, the occurrence of placental remnants is unlikely.

Retention of a succenturiate lobe may catch out the unwary [15]. Due diligence at the time of placental delivery, with careful examination of the placenta and membranes, provides the opportunity to identify an aberrant blood vessel indicating the presence of

Table 9.1 Causes of secondary post-partum or post-abortion haemorrhage (modified from Iraha et al, 2018, permission requested)[8]

	Frequency of occurrence	Imaging features	Treatment	Differential diagnosis
RPOC				
Hypo- to moderate vascular RPOC	Most common	Endometrial echogenic mass with minimum to moderate vascularity	Conservative Medical Surgical removal	Blood clots Endometritis GTD
Hypervascular RPOC	Uncommon	Endometrial echogenic mass with marked vascularity	Surgical removal UAE	GTD UVM Pseudoaneurysm
UVM				
Low-flow UVM (non-AVM*)	Uncommon	Uterine enlargement, large myometrial vessels without arteriovenous shunting	Conservative Balloon tamponade UAE Uterine suture	Vascularised RPOC Pseudoaneurysm
High-flow UVM (true AVM)	Extremely rare	Tortuous, dilated, high-flow myometrial vessels with arteriovenous shunting	UAE Surgical removal of concomitant RPOC following UAE Hysterectomy	Vascularised RPOC Pseudoaneurysm
Pseudoaneurysm of uterine artery	Rare	Smooth-walled sac with high flow	UAE	UVM Vascularised RPOC
GTD	Rare	Hypervascular uterine mass	Surgical removal Chemotherapy Hysterectomy	RPOC UVM

AVM: arteriovenous malformation, GTD: gestational trophoblastic disease, non-AVM: non-arteriovenous vascular malformation, RPOC: retained products of conception, UAE: uterine artery embolisation, UVM: uterine vascular malformation, * probably represents subinvolution of the placental site.

an additional portion of placenta [16]. Further inspection of the uterine cavity is required if this additional portion is absent.

More difficulties arise when removal of the placenta is piecemeal, as will occur with an abnormally adherent or invasive placenta seen with the placenta accreta spectrum disorders, where part or all of the placenta may be incapable of normal separation.

Whatever the circumstances at delivery, inspection of the placenta following its removal and uterine cavity check at CS remain the mainstay of identifying incomplete placental removal, with subsequent active management of suspected retained tissue. It is safest to presume that with piecemeal placental removal, a cotyledon or more may be left inside the uterus and if this is not recognised at the time, it may result in abnormal uterine bleeding (AUB).

A study of secondary PPH in a district general hospital over a three-year period identified associated risk factors following delivery. From the hospital delivered population of over 17 500 women, 132 were admitted with secondary PPH (0.75%). Both recent primary PPH, (odds ratio (OR) 9.3, 95% confidence intervals (CI) 6.2–14.0) and retained placenta requiring manual removal were significant risk factors (OR 3.5, 95% CI 1.6–7.5) [3]. Women who had experienced RPOCs following a previous delivery were also more vulnerable [15].

Some studies found RPOCs in an abnormal uterine cavity in a higher proportion of women than expected, such as a uterine septum or didelphus [17–19]. Previous treatment of a uterine septum did not necessarily prevent RPOCs occurring [18].

9.4 Treatment of Post-Partum Placental Remnants

9.4.1 Expectant Management

Conservative or expectant management is appropriate to consider when the vaginal blood loss is not heavy, there is little evidence of RPOC on USS and Doppler studies demonstrate no or minimal uterine vascularity [2]. Antibiotics are often given in these circumstances on the basis that endometritis is a likely cause of bleeding [6]. There is benefit too in simply monitoring patients over several days, and without the need for them to be resident in hospital, though with clear plans for regular review at defined intervals (see Figure 9.1). Some patients may only require reassurance that what they are experiencing is a variation of normal lochia which will settle spontaneously and without treatment [15]. RPOC may be passed spontaneously, the median duration (and interquartile range) for disappearance on USS for pregnancies ending before 22 weeks' gestation and managed expectantly was 84 days (range 50–111) [20]. Overdiagnosis of RPOC exposes patients to unnecessary trauma by the surgical attempt to remove them. Of note, a significant proportion of women (11%) who undergo surgical treatment do not have RPOC confirmed histologically [7]. There is evidence that expectant management is effective and successful in 50–85% for incomplete miscarriage at less than 13 weeks [21].

9.4.2 Medical Management

Uterotonics, such as the oral synthetic prostaglandin E1 analogue, misoprostol, may be of benefit particularly if the uterus is soft [15]. However, evidence to support their use is limited and investigation with RCTs is recommended [6], and the dose and route of

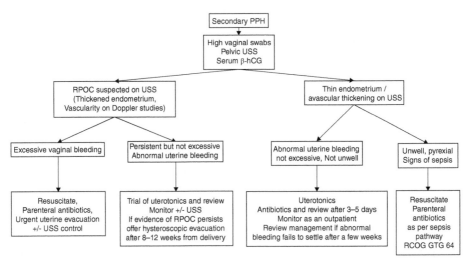

Fig 9.1 Algorithm for the management of postdelivery placental remnants

administration (vaginal versus oral) need to be established. There is evidence that misoprostol is both effective (80–99% across studies) and acceptable following incomplete miscarriage at less than 13 weeks' gestation [21], but this may not be directly relevant to postdelivery circumstances.

9.4.3 Surgical Intervention

Surgical treatment with evacuation of the uterine cavity is traditionally considered to involve dilatation and curettage (D&C) with sharp or blunt curettage or vacuum aspiration. However, hysteroscopic removal (HR) of RPOC is becoming more common with the advantage of precise tissue removal [7, 17, 22]. This is pertinent because only a small portion of the endometrium may be involved with attached RPOC. Blind curettage increases the risk of unnecessary trauma to adjacent, uninvolved endometrium with consequent scarring and adhesion formation [17]. However, there are no RCTs comparing D&C and HR [7], though one randomised study compares two different methods of HR, namely loop resection versus removal with a hysteroscopic tissue removal system (HTRS) [23]. Ultrasound guided D&C is an option to maximise tissue removal, whilst minimising endometrial trauma.

Most studies do not separate treatment of RPOC by duration of the pregnancy following a first or second trimester pregnancy termination or loss from RPOC after birth by vaginal delivery or CS. Complications and outcomes following an early pregnancy loss may differ from after a birth, as indicated by higher incomplete resection rates in the puerperium with a relative risk (RR) of 1.53 (95% CI 1.01–2.32) [7].

A combination of factors may lead to secondary PPH, as may occur when RPOC are present alongside an AVM. Vaginal bleeding may be intermittent, but torrential. In this situation, immediate management with balloon tamponade can help, but interventional arteriography with uterine artery embolisation (UAE) may be necessary [8]. Attention can then be given to removal of the RPOC, or perhaps deferred to a later date when it can be safely achieved without precipitating further heavy bleeding. Hysterectomy is regarded as a last resort when UAE has failed [8].

9.4.3.1 Hysteroscopic Techniques

Cold-loop resection of RPOC was suggested as early as 1997 [24]; this involves using the resection loop as a curette, but without electricity so as not to damage the endometrium. The procedure is often undertaken in the operating theatre under general anaesthetic, partly because of the need to dilate the cervix to 8 or 9 mm, but also because of the ability to increase the intra-uterine pressure to control bleeding from the RPOC, to obtain an adequate view of the tissue, and this is usually painful. However, whichever device is used, the need for cervical dilation depends upon the cervical os diameter, which may be open with retained tissue in the cavity. One circumstance where cervical dilation may be more difficult is when the woman has established breastfeeding and is thus, in a hypoestrogenic state.

RPOC are separated from the endometrium with the loop electrode and then removed from the cavity under direct vision, resulting in the device being removed and reinserted into the cavity multiple times. A specific advantage of using a resectoscope is that electrosurgery can be judiciously applied when a portion of the RPOC is particularly adherent.

An advantage of using a HTRS is that the device remains in the cavity throughout the procedure, with aspiration of RPOC from the cavity, once released from the endometrium, by the mechanically rotating or oscillating cutting device. The outer diameter of HTRSs vary between 5–8 mm; the larger systems are preferable when there is a substantial amount of tissue present to reduce operating time. When the RPOC volume is small (≤ 20 ml) then a smaller system is likely to suffice, with the option of the procedure being undertaken in an office or outpatient setting [25]. Selection of patients for outpatient treatment is advised and limited to those with absent or minimal vascularisation on Doppler studies, an endometrial thickness less than 30 mm and after at least six weeks from the end of the pregnancy (at whatever gestation it occurred) [26]. However, some women may prefer a planned two-stage outpatient procedure rather than a single hospital admission with a general anaesthetic. Such a two-stage procedure will not increase the risk of intra-uterine adhesions (IUAs) [7].

There is also a 5 mm mini-resectoscope available that could be used as a cold loop in an outpatient setting provided the amount of tissue to be removed is small, as noted above.

9.4.3.2 Timing of Surgical Intervention

Timing of the procedure from delivery is important with two studies commenting that hysteroscopic resection should be avoided during the first month after the puerperium and deferred for between two and three months until the uterine cavity is smaller and the RPOC less vascular [19, 23]. This is because of their experiences with short-term complications including sepsis, pulmonary oedema, heavy bleeding, uterine and cervical perforation. Consequently, if earlier surgical intervention is thought necessary because of the heaviness of the vaginal bleeding and RPOCs are thought to be the cause, then the more traditional D&C with digital or vacuum aspiration may be required, and possibly under USS control. However, the uterus remains at risk of perforation and immediate treatment-related heavy vaginal bleeding. The comments made above about the presence and management of an AVM, though extremely rare, should be noted.

9.4.3.3 Effectiveness (complete removal rate)

Studies investigating surgical removal of RPOC frequently combine all gestations of pregnancy and often do not differentiate between them. However, from the subgroup analysis of their review procedures, complete tissue removal was significantly less likely to be achieved post-partum at a single procedure [7]. The pooled complete resection rate after birth (CRR) was reduced to 71% (95% CI 0.41–0.94), compared with 91% (95% CI 0.83–0.96) overall with a RR of 0.75, (95% CI 0.66–0.85). It is likely that post-partum RPOC is more challenging than following an early pregnancy loss because of the larger uterus and the possibility of a greater volume of retained tissue.

In an RCT comparing loop resection and HTRS, both were equally effective at complete tissue removal (95% and 91%, respectively), and though the median operation time in minutes for the HTRS was significantly shorter, 10.0 (interquartile range 5.8–16.4) and 6.2 (4.0–11.2) p = 0.023, both were of short duration [23]. The high CRR is consistent with the results of a systematic review of hysteroscopic resection in which 20 studies with about 2 000 patients were included and where the CRR in a single hysteroscopic procedure was reported as 91% (95% CI 0.83–0.96) [7].

The CRR for D&C is more difficult to establish because of lack of reporting, though one study of 70 patients compared RPOC removal by hysteroscopic loop resection versus D&C, where the procedure was determined by the experience of the surgeon [17]. HR with a single procedure was complete in all 46 women (100%) but 5/24 (21%) women in the D&C group required additional treatment for incomplete tissue removal and this was undertaken hysteroscopically.

The size of the instrument used for tissue removal appears to be more important at achieving a high CRR than the technique or device used [7]. This may simply reflect that a large volume of retained tissue is more difficult to remove completely and takes longer with a smaller device.

Treatment under general anaesthetic was advantageous compared with local or no anaesthetic with a higher CRR (p = 0.01) [7]. Whilst it is convenient for the patient to be treated in an outpatient or office setting, this may not be the most efficient method if a second procedure is required and not necessarily appropriate if the tissue is vascular. However, when only a small amount of tissue is present, complete removal at the time of a diagnostic hysteroscopy during a 'See and Treat' session, may do much to mitigate the anxiety and disruption caused by the retained tissue and its symptoms.

Providing the patient with information about the vascularity of the RPOC, the likely duration of the procedure and probability of a second treatment session will help the patient and clinician when deciding about the treatment venue, when this choice is available. Involving the patient in the decision is important.

9.4.3.4 Short-Term Complications

Immediate complications consist of uterine perforation, cervical laceration, infection with endometritis, mild to heavy vaginal bleeding prompting a blood transfusion and incomplete tissue removal. In a systematic review of hysteroscopic RPOC removal, the complication rate for about 2 000 procedures was 2% (95% CI 0.00–0.04) [7]. There were no evident significant differences in complication rates in the studies that compared different operative techniques, though only one study was an RCT.

9.4.3.5 Longer-Term Outcomes

In the longer term, there are potential consequences for subsequent fertility due to the presence of RPOC, as well as their removal. The development of new IUAs, possibly in response to persisting RPOCs but certainly following trauma to the endometrium during treatment may compromise conception and implantation, or lead to early pregnancy loss or stillbirth [5]. In addition, endometritis may lead to tubal occlusion. Women with IUAs may be asymptomatic, have AUB, hypomenorrhoea or amenorrhoea. Second-look hysteroscopy enables new adhesions to be found and treated and is indicated in symptomatic women and where fertility is of concern. The incidence of IUAs will depend upon the procedure, generally women who re-establish a regular menstrual cycle are not offered further investigation even though asymptomatic women may have IUAs [27, 28].

Outcomes in subsequent pregnancies after postdelivery RPOC removal are difficult to analyse because many of the studies in the reviews do not differentiate between RPOC after an early pregnancy ending and postdelivery [7]. It is unconfirmed whether there are important differences.

Westendorp et al. [5] investigated 50 consecutive women who underwent surgical treatment of RPOC more than 24 hours after either delivery (n = 40) or curettage after previous surgical or medical treatment of an abortion (n = 10) by diagnostic hysteroscopy three months after the procedure. IUAs were found in 20 women (40%), and these were considered of significance in 15 (30%); of note, this rate did not differ between women following delivery and after the ending of an early pregnancy. Risk factors for significant IUAs were lactation, RR 2.6 (95% CI 1.2–5.9 p = 0.04), amenorrhoea, RR 15 (95% CI 2.1–109 p < 0.0001) and dysmenorrhoea, RR 15 (95% CI 1.9–122 p < 0.0001).

In a single retrospective study of 127 women who underwent surgical intervention after a delivery of at least 32 weeks' gestation, 112 were available for follow-up and one third were offered a second-look hysteroscopy either to investigate a menstrual abnormality or confirm cavity integrity [27]. Overall, IUAs were found in 20% of 112 with severe IUAs in 23/37 (62%) women, which is over a fifth of the women followed up. The incidence of IUAs did not vary with the procedure performed (though the study was not an RCT) but was higher in women who underwent a second intervention (9/21, 43%).

A systematic review of mainly cohort studies assessing long-term outcomes following surgical removal of RPOC, after any pregnancy, identified IUAs in 74/330 (22.4%, 95% CI 18.3%–27.2%) women who underwent subsequent hysteroscopy, usually between 3–6 months after surgery [22]. These varied in severity between mild and severe, with significantly more women with moderate adhesions following D&C rather than HR (29/189 vs 5/141 respectively, p < 0.01), though there was no statistical difference for mild and severe adhesions.

The same review sought for outcomes after medical management of RPOC, such as following misoprostol, but found no such studies [22].

Subsequent cumulative conception rates (CCR), pregnancy loss or miscarriage rates (PLR), live birth rates (LBR) and time to conception in women who wish to conceive may indicate the degree of endometrial damage and its consequences. Meta-analysis in a systematic review was compromised by the varied duration of follow-up between studies and was not always recorded [22]. However, CCRs were relatively high with 82.4% (192/233) in the HR group and 81% (119/147) following D&C [22], and a CCR of 87% (95% CI 0.75–0.95) in women following HR [7]. The presence or absence of IUAs was not clear though from the studies. A tendency to earlier conception was found following HR [17, 29], but this has yet to be confirmed by an RCT.

Miscarriage in subsequent pregnancies does not appear to be high with PLR as low as 9–12%, with no apparent difference between HR and D&C [7, 22]. Live birth or ongoing pregnancy rates appear high with pooled LBRs of 71–73.2% [7, 22], and again similar for whichever procedure was undertaken.

There is concern about the effect that delay in performing treatment may have on subsequent reproductive function, particularly if deliberately delayed until 8–12 weeks from delivery. A review of the time from diagnosis (TDT) to complete resection of RPOC [7] found there was no correlation between TDT and completeness of resection or subsequent fertility. This is consistent with the findings of a retrospective study of 75 asymptomatic women undergoing HR of RPOC identified at a routine six-week USS following delivery or miscarriage. They concluded that the time interval from the end of the index pregnancy to RPOC removal did not influence subsequent fertility [28].

9.5 Counselling

The importance of providing women who present with a secondary PPH with an overview of what is likely to be happening and why cannot be overemphasised. The stress for the woman and her partner when a primary PPH happens is recognised [6] and this is the case too when a secondary PPH occurs. Attendance at or admission to hospital in the puerperium is disruptive and unwelcome particularly with a new baby to consider as well; there may also be other children at home.

Care of the patient includes ensuring that they are kept informed about what investigations are indicated, when they will take place and how the results may influence treatment. The initial response will be determined by the severity of the bleeding, with emergency measures if indicated. However, if the blood loss is not so heavy then more time can be taken to establish whether RPOC are present. If the woman is allowed home, then it must be made clear how and when she is to be monitored and how she should seek advice if she has concerns in the meantime.

Communication with the patient and her partner is important, emphasising that definitive removal of intrauterine tissue may be best left for some weeks. They must be reassured too that this is to minimise short-term complications and does not compromise subsequent fertility.

9.6 Summary

Retained placental remnants occur in the puerperium whatever the mode of delivery. Women at risk are those who have had a primary PPH, manual removal of placenta or with a history of RPOCs following a previous delivery. Presentation is commonly with secondary PPH. An USS finding of a vascular echogenic endometrial mass helps differentiate RPOC from a blood clot within the uterine cavity. Initial medical treatment with antibiotics and uterotonics is indicated, especially when the blood loss is not heavy.

There is a range of interventions available, and several may be required depending upon the individual circumstances. Resuscitation with urgent uterine evacuation is indicated if the woman presents with very heavy blood loss and is clinically unstable. With less vaginal blood loss, surgical treatment may be safely deferred for 2–3 months allowing spontaneous resolution, or at least reduction in the size of the uterus and vascularity of the placental remnants.

Hysteroscopic resection of RPOC in an outpatient setting may require more than one procedure for complete removal. A planned two-stage outpatient procedure may be preferable for the woman than a single inpatient session with a general anaesthetic. This does not increase the risk of IUAs developing, unlike an incomplete procedure undertaken blindly by D&C when the persistence of RPOC is unknown. The venue for the procedure may be determined by the volume of tissue to be removed and therefore, the duration of time to complete the procedure. A general anaesthetic in the operating theatre is indicated if the procedure may take over 30 minutes.

Operative complications occur, though are uncommon, and so surgical intervention should be confined to women with scan and Doppler study evidence of RPOCs. A second-look hysteroscopy to assess for incomplete removal of tissue or the presence of IUAs is particularly important for women who wish to conceive, are amenorrhoeic or remain symptomatic with abnormal bleeding. Subsequent reproductive outcomes suggest that most women who wish to conceive will do so successfully, though this may be compromised by IUAs.

Communication with the patient and partner is important to mitigate the stress created by the situation. For example, explanations should be given as to why completion of treatment may be prolonged.

More research is required to establish what treatments are best, with little study to date of medical therapies, the timing of surgical procedures and of the different techniques available.

Clinical Governance Issues

- Exclude GTD if vascular changes on USS with serum β-hCG and histopathology
- Women managed expectantly should have a planned follow-up by a health-care professional (e.g. after two weeks)
- Provide written information to the patient to support oral communication about the management of secondary PPH due to placental remnants, including contact details and indications as to when to make contact
- Consider USS guidance if performing a blind evacuation of the uterus
- HR should be deferred for between two to three months after delivery to avoid complications like uterine perforation and heavy bleeding
- Offer second-look hysteroscopy following surgical intervention

References

1   J. Alexander, P. Thomas and J. Sanghera. Treatments for secondary postpartum haemorrhage. *Cochrane Database of Systematic Reviews (Online)*, (2002), Cd002867.

2   T. Van den Bosch, A. Daeman, D. Van Schoubroeck, et al. Occurrence and outcome of residual trophoblastic tissue. A prospective study. *Journal of Ultrasound in Medicine*, **27** (2008), 357–61.

3   F. Hoveyda and I. Z. MacKenzie.
     Secondary postpartum haemorrhage:
     Incidence, morbidity and current
     management. *BJOG: An International
     Journal of Obstetrics and Gynaecology*,
     108 (2001), 927–30.

4   A. Kamaya, I. Petrovitch, B. Chen, et al.
     Retained products of conception:
     Spectrum of color Doppler findings.
     Journal of Ultrasound in Medicine, **28**
     (2009), 1031–41.

5   I. C. D. Westendorp, W. M. Ankum, B.
     W. J. Mol and J. Vonk. Prevalence of
     Asherman's syndrome after secondary
     removal of placental remnants or a repeat
     curettage for incomplete abortion.
     Human Reproduction, **13** (1998),
     3347–50.

6   E. Mavrides, S. Allard, E. Chandraharan,
     et al. (on behalf of the Royal College of
     Obstetricians and Gynaecologists).
     Prevention and management of
     postpartum haemorrhage. GTG 52.
     *BJOG: An International Journal of
     Obstetrics and Gynaecology*, **124** (2016),
     e106–e149.

7   S. Vitale, J. P. Parry, J. Carugno, et al.
     Surgical and reproductive outcomes after
     hysteroscopic removal of retained
     products of conception: A systematic
     review and meta-analysis. *Journal of
     Minimally Invasive Gynecology*, **28**
     (2021), 204–17.

8   Y. Iraha, M. Okada, M. Toguchi, et al.
     Multimodality imaging in secondary
     postpartum or postabortion hemorrhage:
     Retained products of conception and
     related conditions. *Japanese Journal of
     Radiology*, **36** (2018), 12–22.

9   A. Mulic-Lutvica and O. Axelsson.
     Ultrasound finding of an echogenic mass
     in women with secondary postpartum
     hemorrhage is associated with retained
     placental tissue. *Ultrasound in Obstetrics
     & Gynecology*, **28** (2006), 312–19.

10   N. K. Lee, S. Kim, J. W. Lee, et al.
     Postpartum hemorrhage: Clinical and
     radiologic aspects. *European Journal of
     Radiology*, **74** (2010), 50–9.

11   N. Smorgick, H. Segal, N. Eisenberg, et al.
     Serum b-HCG level in women diagnosed
     as having retained products of
     conception: A prospective cohort study.
     Journal of Minimally Invasive Gynecology,
     29 (2022), 424–28.

12   C. A. Combs, E. L. Murphy and R. K.
     Laros. Factors associated with postpartum
     hemorrhage with vaginal birth. *Obstetrics
     & Gynecology*, **77** (1991), 69–76.

13   F. Urner, R. Zimmermann and A. Krafft.
     Manual removal of the placenta after
     vaginal delivery: An unsolved problem in
     obstetrics. *Journal of Pregnancy*, (2014),
     2746515.

14   S. Greenbaum, T. Wainstock, D. Dukler,
     E. Leron and O. Erez. Underlying
     mechanisms of retained placenta:
     Evidence from a population based cohort
     study. *European Journal of Obstetrics &
     Gynecology and Reproductive Biology*, **216**
     (2017), 12–17.

15   I. A. Babarinsa, R. G. Hayman and T. J.
     Draycott. Secondary post-partum
     haemorrhage: Challenges in evidence-
     based causes and management. *European
     Journal of Obstetrics & Gynecology and
     Reproductive Biology*, **159** (2011), 255–60.

16   NICE CG190. *Intrapartum Care for
     Healthy Women and Babies*. (2019). www
     .nice.org.uk/guidance/cg190/resources/
     intrapartum-care-for-healthy-women-
     and-babies-pdf-35109866447557

17   S. B. Cohen, A. Kalter-Ferber, B. S. Weisz,
     et al. Hysteroscopy may be the method of
     choice for management of residual
     trophoblastic tissue. *Journal of the
     American Association of Gynecologic
     Laparoscopists*, **8** (2001), 199–202.

18   E. Faivre, X. Deffieux, C. Mrazguia, et al.
     Hysteroscopic management of residual
     trophoblastic tissue and reproductive
     outcome: A pilot study. *Journal of
     Minimally Invasive Gynecology*, **16**
     (2009), 487–90.

19   A. Golan, M. Dishi, A. Shalev, et al.
     Operative hysteroscopy to remove
     retained products of conception: Novel
     treatment of an old problem. *Journal of*

Minimally Invasive Gynecology, **18** (2011), 100–3.

20 Y. Wada, H. Hakahashi, H. Suzuki, et al. Expectant management of retained products of conception following abortion: A retrospective cohort study. *European Journal of Obstetrics & Gynecology and Reproductive Biology,* **260** (2021), 1–5.

21 J. P. Neilson, G. M. Gyte, M. Hickey, J. C. Vazquez and L. Dou. Medical treatments for incomplete miscarriage. *Cochrane Database of Systematic Reviews,* (2013), CD007223. https://doi.org/10.1002/14651858.CD007223.pub3

22 A. B. Hooker, H. Aydin, H. A. Brölmann and J. A. Huirne. Long-term complications and reproductive outcome after the management of retained products of conception: A systematic review. *Fertility and Sterility,* **105** (2016), 156–64.

23 T. W. O. Hamerlynck, H. A. A. M. van Vliet, A-S. Beerens, S. Weyers and B. C. Schoot. Hysteroscopic morcellation versus loop resection for removal of placental remnants: A randomized trial. *Journal of Minimally Invasive Gynecology,* **23** (2016), 1172–80.

24 M. Goldenberg, E. Schiff, R. Achiron, S. Lipitz and S. Mashiah. Managing residual trophoblastic tissue: Hysteroscope for directing curettage. *Journal of Reproductive Medicine,* **42** (1997), 26–8.

25 D. Georgiou, A. Tranoulis and T. L. Jackson. Hysteroscopic tissue removal system (MyoSure) for the resection of polyps, submucosal leiomyomas and retained products of conception in an out-patient setting: A single UK institution experience. *European Journal of Obstetrics & Gynecology and Reproductive Biology,* **231** (2018), 147–51.

26 K. Jakopic Macek, M. Blaganje, N. Kenda Suster, K. Drusany Staric and B. Kobal. Office hysteroscopy in removing retained products of conception – a highly successful approach with minimal complications. *Journal of Obstetrics and Gynaecology,* **40** (2020), 1122–6.

27 A. B. Hooker, L. T. Muller, E. Paternotte and A. L. Thurkow. Immediate and long-term complications of delayed surgical management in the postpartum period: A retrospective analysis. *Journal of Maternal-Fetal and Neonatal Medicine,* **28** (2015), 1884–9.

28 M. Tarasov, Y. Z. Burke, D. Stockheim, R. Orvieto and S. B. Cohen. Does the time interval between the diagnosis to hysteroscopic evacuation of retained products of conception affect reproductive outcome. *Archives of Gynecology and Obstetrics,* **302** (2020),1523–8.

29 I. Ben-Ami, Y. Melcer, N. Smorgick, et al. A comparison of reproductive outcomes following hysteroscopic management versus dilatation and curettage of retained products of conception. *International Journal of Gynecology & Obstetrics,* **127** (2014), 86–9.

Gestational Trophoblastic Disease (GTD)

10

Victoria L. Parker, Julia E. Palmer

10.1 Background

Gestational trophoblastic disease (GTD) is an umbrella term for a range of pregnancy-related conditions, with an incidence of 1 in 714 live births [1]. The condition incorporates a spectrum of pre-malignant conditions:

- partial hydatidiform mole (PHM)
- complete hydatidiform mole (CHM), and malignant subtypes (gestational trophoblastic neoplasia (GTN))
- invasive mole
- choriocarcinoma
- placental-site trophoblastic tumour (PSTT)
- epithelioid trophoblastic tumour (ETT)

GTD occurs sporadically at the time of conception with the exact cause yet to be fully characterised [2, 3]. Risk factors for GTD include Asian ethnicity, with an incidence of 1 in 387 compared to 1 in 752 live births for the non-Asian population [4]. Extremes of reproductive age are a particular risk factor for CHM, which affects 1 in 463 pregnancies at age 15 years and 1 in 8 pregnancies in women $\geq$ 50 years [5, 6].

PHM is the most common subtype (1 in 695 pregnancies) and consists of a genetically triploid diandric, monogynic conception, following the fertilisation of one ovum with two sperm (Figure 10.1a). CHM occur less commonly (1 in 945 pregnancies) and are genetically diploid, arising in 75% cases from the fertilisation of an empty ovum with one sperm (monospermic CHM) (Figure 10.1b). The remainder of CHMs are dispermic, occurring when two sperm fertilise an empty ovum (Figure 10.1c) [1-3, 8, 9]. GTN may additionally present after a non-molar pregnancy or post-natally, following the live birth of a healthy infant (1 in 50 000 live births) [1].

Over the last two decades, the rise in the use of ultrasound in early pregnancy units has led to a change in the presentation of GTD. Previously, most molar pregnancies were identified in the second trimester ~16 weeks, whereas nowadays, patients may receive a suspected ultrasound diagnosis as early as 6–8 weeks gestation [10]. PHMs often present later (late first or early second trimester) compared to CHM due to the presence of fetal parts, a gestation sac or intact fetus, which can mimic a viable pregnancy or delayed miscarriage on ultrasound examination [1, 2, 10]. The fetus is characteristically growth restricted and non-viable, with genetic triploidy and congenital abnormalities [1, 9, 11]. Dissimilarly, a CHM contains no fetal parts and generates a characteristically abnormal 'snowstorm' echo appearance on ultrasound, representing the multiple hydropic villi [12].

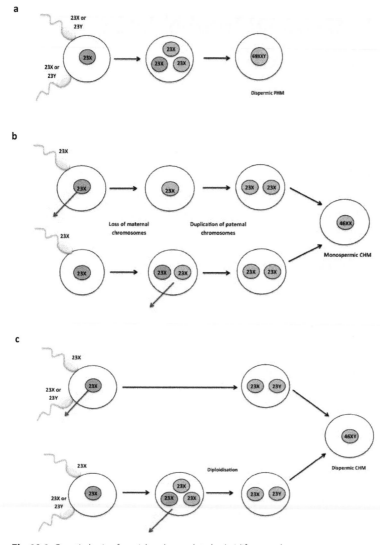

Fig 10.1 Genetic basis of partial and complete hydatidiform moles
(a) **PHM**
(b) **Monospermic CHM**
(c) **Dispermic CHM**

Based on image from Seckl et al. (2013) [7]
Copyright 2013, reproduced with permission from Oxford University Press.
Key: CHM, complete hydatidiform mole; PHM, partial hydatidiform mole.

In the UK, vaginal bleeding is the most common presenting symptom of GTD and GTN, occurring in approximately 60% of cases. Less commonly, women may be large for gestational age due to uterine enlargement (most commonly with CHM); present with hyperemesis gravidarum; or abdominal distention/pain arising from theca lutein ovarian cysts which can occur secondary to ovarian hyperstimulation [1]. Biochemical and clinical hyperthyroidism can also develop in women with high human chorionic gonadotrophin (hCG) levels ($>10^6$ IU/L) [13, 14]. Previously common manifestations of GTD/GTN including pre-eclampsia, anaemia and complications arising from metastatic disease such as eclampsia, haemoptysis and respiratory failure are now extremely rare [10, 15].

GTD is a specialist condition requiring multidisciplinary management, involving medical oncology, radiology, pathology, gynaecology, clinical nurse specialists and counsellors. Women diagnosed with this condition are referred to one of three specialist centres in the United Kingdom, based in Sheffield, London and Dundee, however only Sheffield and London provide treatment for GTN. Women diagnosed with pre-malignant PHM or CHM require surgical uterine evacuation of products of conception and a period of regular monitoring, using serum or urine levels of the GTD tumour marker, hCG. In some cases, the size of fetal parts may preclude the use of surgical evacuation, hence medical evacuation is required and carries an increased risk of incomplete uterine evacuation. Observational data for CHM pregnancies also points to a higher risk of GTN (16-fold) with the use of prostaglandins and oxytocin within a medical evacuation regimen [16]. Women diagnosed with a CHM are monitored for a period of six months following uterine evacuation, yet this may be extended if the hCG takes >56 days to normalise [1]. Follow-up can be shortened for PHM due to the lower rates of malignant conversion; 0.5–1.0% following PHM compared to 13–16% after CHM. During this time, to avoid diagnostic confusion, women are advised not to conceive, as malignant conversion to GTN is most likely to manifest within this initial monitoring period, and presents in a similar way to a new pregnancy, with rising hCG levels.

In the United Kingdom, 8–10% of women develop GTN and require treatment with chemotherapy. Primary chemotherapy choice is guided by the combined International Federation of Gynaecology and Obstetrics (FIGO)/World Health Organization (WHO) scoring system (Table 10.1). This system predicts the risk of single-agent chemotherapy resistance and classifies patients as low risk (total score ≤ 6) versus high risk (total score ≥ 7). Low-risk patients receive primary single-agent chemotherapy whilst high-risk patients are treated with multi-agent chemotherapy from the outset. Women are advised to delay conceiving until 12 months following the completion of their chemotherapy, as the recurrence risk is highest during this time period. Furthermore, delaying conception reduces the risk of fetal teratogenicity arising from chemotherapeutic agents.

10.2 Antenatal

10.2.1 Prior History of GTD or GTN

Pregnant women with a prior history of GTD or GTN who have been discharged from a specialist trophoblastic centre having attained a normal hCG, do not require specialist antenatal management. Such pregnancies can be managed under midwifery-led care.

A study assessing the long-term consequences of pregnancies conceived after completing chemotherapy treatment for invasive mole or choriocarcinoma found no increased risk of miscarriage, fetal anomalies, multiple pregnancy, neonatal or infantile death. Children were followed-up for a maximum of 25 years and had normal growth and development. Furthermore, compared to women who had undergone a

Table 10.1 The combined FIGO/WHO scoring system (FIGO, 2000) [3]

FIGO anatomical stage	
Stage	**Descriptor**
I	Disease confined to the uterus
II	GTN extends outside of the uterus but is limited to the genital structures (adnexae, vagina, broad ligament)
III	GTN extends to the lungs, with or without known genital tract involvement
IV	All other metastatic sites

Modified WHO prognostic classification system, as adapted by FIGO				
	Score			
Risk factor	**0**	**1**	**2**	**4**
Age (years)	<40	≥40	–	–
Antecedent pregnancy	Mole	Abortion	Term	–
Interval months from index pregnancy	<4	4–6	7–12	>12
Pretreatment hCG (IU/L)	$<10^3$	$10^3 – 10^4$	$10^4 – 10^5$	$>10^5$
Largest tumour size including uterus (cm)	<3	3–5	≥5	–
Site of metastases	Lung	Spleen, kidney	Gastrointestinal tract	Liver, brain
Number of metastases	0	1–4	5–8	>8
Previous failed chemotherapy	–	–	Single drug	≥2 drugs

Score ≤ 6 low-risk disease
Score ≥ 7 high-risk disease
KEY: cm, centimetre; FIGO, International Federation of Gynaecology and Obstetrics; hCG, human chorionic gonadotrophin; IU/L, international units per litre; WHO, World Health Organization.

hysterectomy, women who had a subsequent pregnancy displayed no increased risk of disease relapse or death secondary to disease [17].

10.2.2 Early Pregnancy in GTD or GTN

Women who have become pregnant *prior* to discharge from a specialist trophoblastic centre who are undergoing active follow-up for GTD or GTN will require multidisciplinary input to differentiate between persistent or recurrent trophoblastic disease and a new, non-molar pregnancy. This will be coordinated by the specialist trophoblastic centre and will predominantly involve radiologists and medical oncologists with surveillance using serial hCG, ultrasound or MRI to reach a diagnosis. Typically, a diagnosis can usually be established by 8–12 weeks' gestation. If a new, viable pregnancy is confirmed, women undergoing surveillance for GTD (who have not required chemotherapy treatment) can be managed under midwifery-led care. Amongst GTD patients who conceived within one year of a PHM or CHM diagnosis, a 71–75% live birth rate and 22% spontaneous miscarriage rate has been observed [18, 19], equivalent to the outcomes of women that had completed their hCG follow-up (77% term birth rate) [20, 21].

However, women who required chemotherapy for GTN, with an interval <12 months after the completion of chemotherapy treatment, should be booked under consultant-led care to discuss the data surrounding such pregnancies and their outcomes. Women should be informed that current knowledge is based on the UK cohort of approximately 500 early pregnant patients, incorporating data from two studies involving n = 230 [22] and n = 255 patients [23]. The discussion should incorporate the following areas:

10.2.2.1 Termination of pregnancy

Termination of pregnancy rates tend to be higher amongst women receiving multi-agent high-risk treatment as the individual feels less physically well, whereas low-risk chemotherapy treatment is generally well tolerated. Furthermore, in low-risk disease, obstetricians and medical oncologists are likely to be more comfortable with continuing the pregnancy under close antenatal surveillance. This would involve a detailed anatomy scan to exclude fetal anomalies and serial ultrasound growth scans throughout the pregnancy, each examining the placenta closely for areas of concern.

10.2.2.2 Miscarriage

Miscarriage rates are higher amongst women receiving treatment for high-risk (18%) as compared to low-risk (8–10%) GTN [22, 24], though the risk is comparable to the miscarriage rate for the general population [23].

10.2.2.3 Fetal anomalies and stillbirth

Rates of fetal anomalies in GTN patients who became pregnant early (1.3–2.5%) are similar to those of the general population (1.6%) [19, 22]. Stillbirth rates (1%) are also in line with those of the general population (0.7%) [22, 23].

10.2.2.4 Live birth rates

Live birth rates at term are comparable in women with an early pregnancy (69–76%) [18, 19, 22–24] versus those who wait >12 months following the completion of chemotherapy treatment. Live birth rates are also in line with those of the general population, highlighting that GTN does not affect subsequent reproductive outcomes [20, 25].

10.2.2.5 Relapse

The risk of disease relapse is not increased amongst women who become pregnant within 12 months of completing treatment [22, 23]. In fact, two studies have shown that relapse rates amongst early pregnant patients are lower (1.7%) compared to patients who did not conceive early (5% and 5.5%). This holds for patients with both low-risk (2%) and high-risk disease (2.5%) [22]. Within this study of 230 early pregnant women, four out of five that relapsed intrapartum delivered a healthy term baby, with one woman requiring early delivery at 36 weeks due to symptomatic advanced disease (multiple pulmonary metastases). All five women were cured following post-partum treatment with combination chemotherapy +/− hysterectomy and remained disease free within a 5–30-year follow-up period [22].

10.2.2.6 Risk of second molar pregnancy

Early pregnancy does not appear to increase the risk of having a second molar pregnancy (1%) versus a baseline 0.7% risk in women who have experienced one molar pregnancy [19, 22, 23].

10.2.3 Twin Pregnancy with a Hydatidiform Mole and Viable Coexistent Fetus

Twin pregnancies involving a hydatidiform mole and a viable coexistent fetus are a rare form of GTD, occurring in 1:20, 000–1:100,000 pregnancies [26, 27]. A viable fetus may coexist with either a PHM or CHM, yet the former is less common due to the high risk of miscarriage with a triploid fetus. Suspected cases should be referred to a specialist fetal medicine and trophoblastic disease centre for multidisciplinary management to help distinguish between the different types of twin mole and viable pregnancy. These include:

- dizygotic diamniotic twin pregnancy with a CHM and coexistent viable, live fetus of diploid karyotype
- dizygotic diamniotic twin pregnancy with a PHM and coexistent viable, live fetus of diploid karyotype
- a monozygotic, diamniotic twin pregnancy with a PHM and live triploid fetus [28]

If uncertainties arise on imaging, prenatal invasive testing for fetal karyotype is often recommended to determine whether the live pregnancy is of diploid or triploid karyotype, as this will affect prognosis and management decisions [1]. A further important differential diagnosis for prognostic and management purposes includes placental mesenchymal dysplasia, a rare condition involving an enlarged placenta, congested and dilated vessels within the chorionic plate but crucially, no evidence of trophoblastic proliferation [29]. This condition involves specific antenatal complications, yet importantly does not carry the risk of developing into GTN, and so elective termination would be unnecessary in most cases [30].

A diagnosis of twin pregnancy involving a hydatidiform mole and viable coexistent fetus is typically reached at 12–14 weeks gestation and patients must be counselled appropriately. Based on the potential risks involved, some patients may wish to electively terminate the pregnancy, whilst others may continue, acknowledging the high intrapartum and post-partum complication rates.

10.2.3.1 Misdiagnosis

Given the rare nature of twin pregnancies with a mole and viable coexistent fetus, misdiagnosis is not uncommon. CHM with a viable coexistent fetus may be reported as a subchorionic haematoma on first trimester ultrasound imaging (50% occurrence) [31], highlighting the need for expert review. In a UK study at the Sheffield Trophoblastic Centre, only 30% of referred cases of twin hydatidiform mole with viable fetus were confirmed on expert histopathological review, highlighting the importance of gaining a second opinion from a specialist team [32].

Table 10.2 Risk of antenatal complications in twin pregnancies involving a hydatidiform mole and viable coexistent fetus

Complication	Occurrence (%)	Reference
Vaginal bleeding	17	[33]
	21	[26]
	60	[34]
	88	[35] [36]
Hyperthyroidism	15	[34]
	28	[26]
Hyperemesis gravidarum	7	[34]
	38	[35]
Preterm birth	20	[33]
	33	[26]
Spontaneous abortion/Intra-uterine death	21	[26]
	36	[31]
	44	[32]
	58	[27]
Pre-eclampsia	28	[33] [26]
	50	[34]

10.2.3.2 Complications

Twin pregnancies with a hydatidiform mole and viable coexistent fetus are at higher risk of antenatal complications, greater than those usually anticipated in twin pregnancies involving two viable fetuses. A comprehensive discussion should take place, covering potential complications including vaginal bleeding, miscarriage, hyperemesis gravidarum, thromboembolic events, fetal growth restriction and preterm birth. Table 10.2 summarises the reported risks of these complications within the published literature. Preterm birth occurs in up to one third of cases, with studies reporting delivery at an average gestational age of 26 [26], 31 [31] and 35 weeks [27, 33]. Rates of spontaneous abortion and intra-uterine fetal death are also high, occurring in 5% [33], 21% [26] and 43% [27] of twin molar and coexistent viable pregnancies at a gestational age ≤24 weeks. Rates are similar at >24 weeks gestation, ranging between 5% [33] and 15% [27].

Pre-eclampsia has been reported in 20–28% of such twin pregnancies [26, 33, 34], yet in a UK cohort study, severe pre-eclampsia prompting termination of pregnancy <24 weeks or early preterm delivery <30 weeks was observed in only 4% and 2% of twin CHM and viable coexistent fetus pregnancies, respectively [27]. Most cases present intrapartum, however post-partum presentation has also been reported [26].

It is disputed whether the presence of complications such as vaginal bleeding and pre-eclampsia is associated with a higher risk of developing GTN. To date, one study is in favour [33] and another in disagreement [26].

10.2.3.3 Termination of Pregnancy

Due to the high rate of antenatal, intrapartum and post-partum complications, termination of pregnancy should be discussed. Studies from different countries have reported variable termination rates, which may reflect the level of expertise in managing such cases. For example, an Italian study documented a 15% termination rate, with 25% of women electively terminating before 14 weeks and 6% between 15–22 weeks [31]. Rates in the UK, Japan and France appear to be higher. A UK study reported that 34% of pregnancies involving a twin mole and coexistent viable fetus were terminated; 73% of which occurred at <14 weeks gestation [27]. In a Japanese study, 62% terminated the pregnancy; 28% of which electively terminated at <16 weeks [33], with similar rates in France; 57% overall termination rate, 43% of which terminated at ≤16 weeks [26].

10.2.3.4 Live Birth Rates

Live birth rates for the viable fetus in a twin CHM pregnancy are variable, ranging between 23–55% (Table 10.3). Logistic regression analysis has suggested that the continuation of pregnancy and attainment of fetal viability is more likely if the following conditions are satisfied:

- an absence of specific antenatal complications including pregnancy-induced hypertension, hyperthyroidism and hyperemesis gravidarum
- an initial serum hCG level < 400,000 mIU/mL

This model generated an area under the curve of 0.74 using a receiver operating characteristics curve [34].

10.2.3.5 Risk of Developing GTN

Previous literature has raised concerns regarding a higher incidence of GTN amongst patients with a twin pregnancy involving a hydatidiform mole, yet there is debate in the literature regarding the exact rates. Studies from Japan (n = 18) [33], France (n = 14) [26], and the USA ((n = 7) [37] & (n = 22)[38]) are broadly consistent, reporting that

Table 10.3 Reported live birth rates in twin pregnancies involving a hydatidiform mole and viable coexistent fetus

Live birth rate (%)	Study details	Reference
23	Japanese study, n = 18	[33]
33	French study, n = 14	[26]
38	UK study, n = 77	[27]
45	Italian study, n = 13	[31]
55	UK study, n = 9	[32]

50–55% cases of twin pregnancies including a CHM and coexistent fetus progress to GTN [26, 33]. One study from the USA reported higher GTN rates of 63% (n = 8) [36].

Meanwhile, a UK study (n = 9) quoted GTN rates of 33% [32], with Dutch (n = 8) [35] and Danish studies (n = 8) [35] revealing a similar, 25% risk of developing GTN. A literature review of 206 cases found 37% developed GTN [34]. However, the largest cohort study to date, involving 77 UK patients has shown rates of GTN following a twin CHM pregnancy (15%) [27] to be equivalent to those following a singleton CHM pregnancy (16%) [1, 2].

Despite these differences, the likelihood of developing GTN is equivalent in women who terminate (16%) or continue with the pregnancy (21%) [27], and is independent of gestational age at the time of termination or delivery [26, 33]. Once again, the risk of GTN is in line with that following a singleton CHM pregnancy (16%) [1, 2]. Interestingly, the risk of GTN appears to be lower following a live birth (23%) compared to pregnancies which have an adverse perinatal outcome (50%) [34]. Reassuringly, all patients achieved a cure with chemotherapy alone [26, 27, 33]. In a UK study, 73% of women required only single-agent chemotherapy, with no maternal deaths and all women were disease free 12 years following diagnosis [27]. Similarly, in one French and one Dutch study, 86% [26] and 100% of women [35] were cured with single-agent chemotherapy [26]. Only one study, which reported outright high rates of GTN, documented a predominant requirement for multi-agent therapy in 60% of women [36].

Ovarian stimulation certainly increases the risk of twin pregnancy. However, there are insufficient data regarding whether ovarian stimulation is a risk factor for developing GTN in twin pregnancies with CHM. Only one study has reported on this outcome measure, with all four patients who received ovarian stimulation with either clomiphene or human gonadotrophins progressing to GTN [26].

10.3 Intrapartum

10.3.1 Prior History of GTD/GTN and Early Pregnant GTD Patients
There are no specific intrapartum considerations for these patient groups. Such women are suitable for intrapartum midwifery-led care.

10.3.2 Early Pregnant GTN Patients
Providing that no concerns have been highlighted in the antenatal period, including fetal anomaly or serial growth ultrasound scans, women can receive intrapartum midwifery-led care. Antenatal concerns with fetal imaging or pregnancy-induced conditions (e.g. obstetric cholestasis, pre-eclampsia) should be managed according to the unit's standard intrapartum pathways, which will determine the requirement for consultant-led care, intrapartum monitoring and guide to a suitable place of delivery.

10.3.3 Twin Pregnancy with a Hydatidiform Mole and Viable Coexistent Fetus
Such pregnancies are at high risk of antenatal complications (e.g. pre-eclampsia, intra-uterine growth restriction) as discussed above and therefore should be managed under consultant-led care, delivering in hospital with continuous electro-fetal monitoring

intrapartum. Due to the higher risk of vaginal bleeding including post-partum haemor-rhage, it is advised that these women have pre-emptive intrapartum intravenous access and receive active management of the third stage of labour.

10.4 Post-Partum

10.4.1 Prior History of GTD and Early Pregnant GTD Patients

There are no specific post-partum considerations for these patient groups. The risk of recurrent GTD in this cohort is low (1:4,110 pregnancy events), therefore a post-natal urine sample or histological examination of the pregnancy tissue is not required [39]. Breastfeeding is safe in this patient group.

10.4.2 Prior History of GTN and Early Pregnant GTN Patient

Women who have a history of chemotherapy treatment for GTN have a risk of recurrent GTD (1:337 pregnancy events) in all subsequent pregnancies. Women should notify the specialist trophoblastic centre of their pregnancy event and undergo post-pregnancy screening for recurrent GTD. Specifically, hCG levels should be measured on a urine sample sent 6–10 weeks following the end of the pregnancy event. Histological examination of the pregnancy tissue however is not required. Breastfeeding is safe in this patient group.

10.4.3 Twin Pregnancy with CHM

Such women have a higher risk of post-partum haemorrhage and should be advised to receive active management of the third stage of labour to minimise blood loss. Care should be taken to ensure the placenta is complete and sent for histological examination to categorically confirm the diagnosis.

There is no consensus on the post-partum management of this patient group, largely due to the rare nature of this condition. The largest published cohort study (n = 77cases) suggests that rates of GTN are equivalent to those following a singleton pregnancy (15%); however, due to variations in reported rates (25–55% risk of GTN), it would be prudent to advise post-partum hCG screening in this group. Histological examination of the pregnancy tissue is not required. Breastfeeding is safe in this patient group.

10.4.4 Contraception

In all patient groups, the combined oral contraceptive pill can be used post-partum, even if hCG levels remain elevated. Progesterone containing contraceptives do not increase the risk of GTN and are safe to use [40]. Intra-uterine contraceptive coils should not be inserted at the time of delivery/uterine evacuation or indeed until hCG levels have returned to normal due to the risk of uterine perforation and bleeding [41]. This includes the use of copper intra-uterine devices for emergency contraceptive purposes. Oral emergency contraception, involving levonorgestrel or ulipristal acetate can be used safely.

10.4.5 Rare Presentations of GTN

A diagnosis of post-partum choriocarcinoma should be considered, although rare (1:50, 000 live births) [10] in women presenting with persistent post-partum bleeding following the delivery of a healthy infant, particularly when there is evidence of retained products of conception on ultrasound imaging. Vaginal bleeding is the most common symptom of this condition, occurring in ~60% cases. Much rarer presentations include respiratory (haemoptysis, shortness of breath) or neurological symptoms [15]. All tissue, whether spontaneously or surgically evacuated, should be sent for histological examination and a serum hCG level should be measured, with abnormally high hCG levels being suggestive of GTN. For reference, serum hCG levels should have normalised by six weeks post-partum.

10.5 Conclusions

GTD is a rare, but important condition, which obstetricians may encounter every one to two years. Women affected by this condition are often understandably anxious regarding subsequent pregnancies, and it is therefore important that obstetricians not only acknowledge this, but also counsel patients accurately and signpost them to appropriate resources. The UK is fortunate in having centralised care for women diagnosed with GTD, and the three specialist trophoblastic centres in Sheffield, London and Dundee can be contacted for expert input and advice. Indeed, for certain cases (early pregnancy in patients diagnosed with GTN or a twin pregnancy with a complete mole and viable coexistent fetus), multidisciplinary management involving the obstetrician and specialist trophoblastic centre should be undertaken. Antenatal, intrapartum and post-partum management is dependent on whether women had a prior diagnosis of GTD or GTN requiring chemotherapy treatment, and it is essential to establish this information as early as possible. Fortunately, the majority of women with a prior history of GTD or GTN go on to have a healthy, viable pregnancy with live birth rates equivalent to the general population.

Clinical Governance Issues

- Women with a history of GTD or GTN should receive detailed pre-conception counselling in a multidisciplinary setting, ideally involving both obstetricians and specialists from a specialist trophoblastic centre
- Women with a prior history of GTD or GTN that have completed treatment do not require specialist antenatal management and can be managed under midwifery-led care
- Women who become pregnant early before completing hCG monitoring for GTD or GTN must be managed in a multidisciplinary setting by a specialist trophoblastic centre to determine whether the pregnancy is viable, represents persistent trophoblastic disease (GTN) or disease recurrence
- Following a diagnosis of GTD, if a new viable pregnancy is confirmed prior to the completion of hCG monitoring, outcomes are favourable. Live birth and miscarriage rates are equivalent to women who have completed their follow-up prior to conceiving. Women can be managed under midwifery-led care
- Following a diagnosis of GTN, women who become pregnant 'early' <12 months from completing chemotherapy treatment have good outcomes. Live birth rates are equivalent to women waiting >12 months to conceive, with no increased risk of relapse or second molar pregnancy. Miscarriage, stillbirth and congenital anomaly rates are in line with the general population

- Obstetricians and trophoblastic disease specialists are more comfortable in managing early pregnancies following low as opposed to high-risk GTN. Termination of pregnancy may be considered
- Women with a twin pregnancy involving a hydatidiform mole and a coexistent viable fetus are at increased risk of antenatal, intrapartum and post-partum complications and should be counselled accordingly and monitored closely
- Complications of twin hydatidiform mole and coexistent viable pregnancies include vaginal bleeding, hyperemesis gravidarum, hyperthyroidism, pre-eclampsia, thromboembolic events, fetal growth restriction and preterm birth
- The live birth rates for women with a twin molar and viable pregnancy lie between 23–55%. Termination of pregnancy should be discussed
- Post-partum, women who have a prior history of GTD or early pregnant GTD patients do not require hCG screening 6–10 weeks following delivery due to the low risk of recurrent GTD (occurs in 1:4 110 pregnancy events)
- Post-partum, women with a prior history of GTN, early GTN or a twin pregnancy with a hydatidiform mole and coexistent viable fetus should have a post-partum hCG sample 6–10 weeks following delivery to exclude recurrent GTD (occurs in 1:337 pregnancy events)
- Histological examination of the pregnancy tissue is not required in any patient group (prior history of GTD, GTN, early pregnant GTD or GTN patients, or twin hydatidiform mole and coexistent fetus)
- Oestrogen and progesterone containing contraception can be safely used in all women with a history of GTD/GTN, even if the hCG levels remain elevated
- Intra-uterine contraceptive devices should not be inserted at the time of delivery/ evacuation or for emergency contraceptive purposes until the hCG has normalised, due to the risk of bleeding and uterine perforation
- Oral emergency contraception, including levonorgestrel or ulipristal acetate can be used safely
- Post-partum choriocarcinoma after a live birth (1:50, 000 live births) should be considered in women who present with persistent vaginal bleeding following the delivery of a healthy infant
- A diagnosis of post-partum choriocarcinoma can be confirmed by raised serum hCG levels and on histological examination of any evacuated tissue
- Breastfeeding is safe in all patient groups

References

1 J. A. Tidy, M. Seckl and B. Hancock (on behalf of the Royal College of Obstetricians and Gynaecologists). Management of gestational trophoblastic disease: Green-top Guideline No. 38 – June 2020. *BJOG: An International Journal of Obstetrics and Gynaecology*, **128** (2021), e1–e27.

2 M. J. Seckl, N. J. Sebire and R. S. Berkowitz. Gestational trophoblastic disease. *Lancet*, **376** (2010), 717–29.

3 H. Y. S. Ngan, M. J. Seckl, R. S. Berkowitz, et al. Diagnosis and management of gestational trophoblastic disease: 2021 update. *International Journal of Gynecology & Obstetrics*, **155** (2021), 86–93.

4 B. W. Tham, J. E. Everard, J. A. Tidy, D. Drew and B. W. Hancock. Gestational trophoblastic disease in the Asian population of Northern England and North Wales. *BJOG: An International Journal of Obstetrics and Gynaecology*, **110** (2003), 555–9.

5   P. M. Savage, A. Sita-Lumsden, S. Dickson, et al. The relationship of maternal age to molar pregnancy incidence, risks for chemotherapy and subsequent pregnancy outcome. *Journal of Obstetrics and Gynaecology,* 33 (2013), 406–11.

6   A. A. Gockley, A. Melamed, N. T. Joseph, et al. The effect of adolescence and advanced maternal age on the incidence of complete and partial molar pregnancy. *Gynecologic Oncology,* 140 (2016), 470–3.

7   M. J. Seckl, N. J. Sebire, R. A. Fisher, et al. Gestational trophoblastic disease: ESMO Clinical Practice Guidelines for diagnosis, treatment and follow-up. *Annals of Oncology: Official Journal of the European Society for Medical Oncology/ESMO,* 24 (2013), vi39–50.

8   M. C. Choi, C. Lee, H. O Smith and S. J. Kim. Epidemiology. In B. W. Hancock, M. J. Seckl and R. S. Berkowitz, eds., *Gestational Trophoblastic Disease.* (2015). https://isstd.org/gtd-book.html

9   H. Dearden and R. Fisher. Genetics. In *Gestational Trophoblastic Disease.* (2015). https://isstd.org/gtd-book.html

10   V. Parker and J. A. Tidy. Current management of gestational trophoblastic disease. *Obstetrics, Gynaecology & Reproductive Medicine,* 31 (2021), 21–9.

11   R. S. Berkowitz and D. P. Goldstein. Current management of gestational trophoblastic diseases. *Gynecologic Oncology,* 112 (2009), 654–62.

12   C. B. Benson, D. R. Genest, M. R. Bernstein, et al. Sonographic appearance of first trimester complete hydatidiform moles. *Ultrasound in Obstetrics and Gynecology,* 16 (2000), 188–91.

13   S. M. Amir, R. Osathanondh, R. S. Berkowitz and D. P. Goldstein. Human chorionic gonadotropin and thyroid function in patients with hydatidiform mole. *American Journal of Obstetrics and Gynecology,* 150 (1984), 723–8.

14   L. Walkington, J. Webster, B. W. Hancock, J. Everard and R. E. Coleman. Hyperthyroidism and human chorionic gonadotrophin production in gestational trophoblastic disease. *British Journal of Cancer,* 104 (2011), 1665–9.

15   E. Diver, T. May, R. Vargas, et al. Changes in clinical presentation of postterm choriocarcinoma at the New England Trophoblastic Disease Center in recent years. *Gynecologic Oncology,* 130 (2013), 483–6.

16   J. A. Tidy, A. M. Gillespie, N. Bright, et al. Gestational trophoblastic disease: A study of mode of evacuation and subsequent need for treatment with chemotherapy. *Gynecologic Oncology,* 78 (2000), 309–12.

17   H. Z. Song, P. C. Wu, Y. E. Wang, X. Y. Yang and S. Y. Dong. Pregnancy outcomes after successful chemotherapy for choriocarcinoma and invasive mole: Long-term follow-up. *American Journal of Obstetrics and Gynecology,* 158 (1988), 538–45.

18   Z. S. Tuncer, M. R. Bernstein, D. P. Goldstein, K. H. Lu and R. S. Berkowitz. Outcome of pregnancies occurring within 1 year of hydatidiform mole. *Obstetrics and Gynecology,* 94 (1999), 588–90.

19   R. S. Berkowitz, Z. S. Tuncer, M. R. Bernstein and D. P. Goldstein. Management of gestational trophoblastic diseases: Subsequent pregnancy experience. *Seminars in Oncology,* 27 (2000), 678–85.

20   R. S. Berkowitz, S. S. Im, M. R. Bernstein and D. P. Goldstein. Gestational trophoblastic disease. Subsequent pregnancy outcome, including repeat molar pregnancy. *The Journal of Reproductive Medicine,* 43 (1998), 81–6.

21   J. H. Kim, D. C. Park, S. N. Bae, S. E. Namkoong and S. J. Kim. Subsequent reproductive experience after treatment for gestational trophoblastic disease. *Gynecologic Oncology,* 71 (1998), 108–12.

22   S. P. Blagden, M. A. Foskett, R. A. Fisher, et al. The effect of early pregnancy following chemotherapy on disease relapse and foetal outcome in women treated for gestational trophoblastic tumours. *British Journal of Cancer,* 86 (2002), 26–30.

23   J. Williams, D. Short, L. Dayal, et al. Effect of early pregnancy following chemotherapy on disease relapse and fetal outcome in women treated for gestational trophoblastic neoplasia. *The Journal of Reproductive Medicine,* 59 (2014), 248–54.

24 Z. S. Tuncer, M. R. Bernstein, D. P. Goldstein and R. S. Berkowitz. Outcome of pregnancies occurring before completion of human chorionic gonadotropin follow-up in patients with persistent gestational trophoblastic tumor. *Gynecologic Oncology*, **73** (1999), 345–7.

25 R. P. Woolas, M. Bower, E. S. Newlands, et al. Influence of chemotherapy for gestational trophoblastic disease on subsequent pregnancy outcome. *British Journal of Obstetrics and Gynaecology*, **105** (1998), 1032–5.

26 J. Massardier, F. Golfier, D. Journet, et al. Twin pregnancy with complete hydatidiform mole and coexistent fetus: Obstetrical and oncological outcomes in a series of 14 cases. *European Journal of Obstetrics, Gynecology, and Reproductive Biology*, **143** (2009), 84–7.

27 N. J. Sebire, M. Foskett, F. J. Paradinas, et al. Outcome of twin pregnancies with complete hydatidiform mole and healthy co-twin. *Lancet*, **359** (2002), 2165–6.

28 K. Gupta, B. Venkatesan, M. Kumaresan and T. Chandra. Early detection by ultrasound of partial hydatidiform mole with a coexistent live fetus. *World Medical Journal*, **114** (2015), 208–11.

29 C. Marusik, C. Frykholm, K. Ericson, J. Wikström and O. Axelsson. Diagnosis of placental mesenchymal dysplasia with magnetic resonance imaging. *Ultrasound in Obstetrics & Gynecology*, **49** (2017), 410–2.

30 L. M. Ernst. Placental mesenchymal dysplasia. *Journal of Fetal Medicine*, **2** (2015), 127–33.

31 V. Giorgione, P. Cavoretto, G. Cormio, et al. Prenatal diagnosis of twin pregnancies with complete hydatidiform mole and coexistent normal fetus: A series of 13 cases. *Gynecologic and Obstetric Investigation*, **82** (2017), 404–9.

32 B. W. Hancock, K. Martin, C. A. Evans, J. E. Everard and M. Wells. Twin mole and viable fetus: The case for misdiagnosis. *The Journal of Reproductive Medicine*, **51** (2006), 825–8.

33 H. Matsui, S. Sekiya, T. Hando, N. Wake and Y. Tomoda. Hydatidiform mole coexistent with a twin live fetus: A national collaborative study in Japan. *Human Reproduction*, **15** (2000), 608–11.

34 M. Suksai, C. Suwanrath, O. Kor-Anantakul, et al. Complete hydatidiform mole with co-existing fetus: Predictors of live birth. *European Journal of Obstetrics, Gynecology, and Reproductive Biology*, **212** (2017), 1–8.

35 I. Niemann, L. Sunde and L. K. Petersen. Evaluation of the risk of persistent trophoblastic disease after twin pregnancy with diploid hydatidiform mole and coexisting normal fetus. *American Journal of Obstetrics and Gynecology*, **197** (2007), e1–5.

36 M. A. Steller, D. R. Genest, M. R. Bernstein, et al. Natural history of twin pregnancy with complete hydatidiform mole and coexisting fetus. *Obstetrics and Gynecology*, **83** (1994), 35–42.

37 D. A. Fishman, L. A. Padilla, P. Keh, et al. Management of twin pregnancies consisting of a complete hydatidiform mole and normal fetus. *Obstetrics and Gynecology*, **91** (1998), 546–50.

38 M. A. Steller, D. R. Genest, M. R. Bernstein, et al. Clinical features of multiple conception with partial or complete molar pregnancy and coexisting fetuses. *The Journal of Reproductive Medicine*, **39** (1994), 147–54.

39 K. E. Earp, B. W. Hancock, D. Short, et al. Do we need post-pregnancy screening with human chorionic gonadotrophin after previous hydatidiform mole to identify patients with recurrent gestational trophoblastic disease? *European Journal of Obstetrics, Gynecology, and Reproductive Biology*, **234** (2019), 117–9.

40 H. L. F. F. Costa and P. Doyle. Influence of oral contraceptives in the development of post-molar trophoblastic neoplasia: A systematic review. *Gynecologic Oncology*, **100** (2006), 579–85.

41 The Faculty of Sexual and Reproductive Healthcare. *Contraception After Pregnancy, FSRH Guideline*. (2020). www.fsrh.org/documents/contraception-after-pregnancy-guideline-january-2017/

11 Female Genital Mutilation

Juliet Albert

11.1 Introduction

11.1.1 Definition

The World Health Organization (WHO) defines female genital mutilation (FGM) as: 'the partial or total removal of, or injury to, the external female genitalia for non-medical reasons'[1] and estimates that more than 200 million girls and women alive today have undergone FGM [1].

FGM is recognised as a form of gender-based violence and a violation of the human rights of women and girls [2] and in 2015, ending FGM was made one of the United Nations Sustainable Development Goals [3]. There are no health benefits, and the practice is associated with a range of physical and psychological complications. Treatment of the health complications of FGM in 27 high prevalence countries is estimated to cost 1.4 billion USD per year [1]. FGM is a global public health concern and is an important health-care challenge in countries such as the UK with large diaspora communities. The practice is illegal in at least 59 countries including the UK.

11.1.2 History

FGM is believed to have existed since the fifth century BC [4, 5]. The phrase 'pharaonic circumcision' is commonly used by East African women to describe Type 3 FGM, suggesting an origin in ancient Egypt.

Although FGM was first reported in parts of Africa it has since been discovered amongst communities in Eastern Europe, Latin America, South-Eastern Asia and the Middle East and among diaspora communities in Western Europe, North America and Australia. More recently, FGM cases have also been identified in Yemen, Syria, Northern Iraq, amongst Kurdish populations in Russia, in Dawoodi Bohra Muslim communities in Pakistan and India, in Colombia and Peru and parts of Indonesia, Malaysia and Papa New Guinea [6]. There is clearly no one homogenous FGM practising community, but a variety of diverse people, customs, cultures and traditions and it is this complexity that has contributed to the endurance of the practice.

11.1.3 Why Is FGM Practised?

Various social and cultural factors are cited as being the reason why FGM is performed. Table 11.1 lists some myths that are used to justify FGM.

FGM is often thought to be a Muslim practice and the phrase 'sunnah' is sometimes used to describe Type 1 and Type 2 FGM implying a religious obligation. However, no

Table 11.1 Common myths used to justify FGM

Custom & tradition	Family honour
Religion	Preparation and eligibility for marriage and right to inherit
Cut genitals perceived as 'clean' and 'beautiful'	Enhancing fertility
Virginity & chastity	A sense of belonging to the group or conversely a fear of social exclusion
Increasing sexual pleasure for men	Peer pressure
Social pressure/norms	Preservation of virginity prior to marriage and ensure fidelity after marriage
Clitoris seen as masculine and so removal increases perceived femininity	Rite of passage from childhood to womanhood
Male coercion and control	Reducing female promiscuity

religious texts prescribe the practice. Furthermore, FGM has been found amongst Ethiopian Falasha Jews as well as in many Christian communities such as in Egypt, Eritrea, Nigeria and elsewhere.

Often village elders have passed down traditional beliefs which perpetuate the practice. For example, the belief that the clitoris will continue growing if it is not cut and that this could render the female daughter infertile or lead to the death of a child during childbirth [7]. There remains a lot of secrecy surrounding the practice and women have sometimes been told that they will die if they tell anyone that they have undergone FGM [7].

11.1.4 Incidence

A UNICEF report highlighted in 2021 that: 'the practice of FGM has been declining over the last three decades...but the pace (of change) has been uneven'[8].

Although FGM is less common in countries where it was historically universal, for example Egypt, Eritrea, Sierra Leone and Kenya; in other countries such as Somalia, Guinea and Mali little has changed over the last 30 years [6]. Nevertheless, despite aims to achieve gender equality, empower women and girls and eradicate FGM by 2030, [3] overall it is estimated that the prevalence of FGM may rise over the next 15 years as the world population grows [9]

FGM is performed on babies as well as grown women but is most common in girls aged 6–15 years [8]. Population Council research carried out from 2015 to 2019 in Somaliland, Kenya, Ethiopia and Senegal found that FGM is being performed on younger girls, in less public ceremonies, there may be less Type 3 and it is increasingly carried out by health-care professionals [10]. This growing medicalisation of FGM is of great concern[11].

Table 11.2 WHO classification of FGM types

FGM type	Description
Type 1	Partial or total removal of the clitoral glans and/or the prepuce. Sometimes known as clitoridectomy **Type Ia**, removal of the clitoral hood or prepuce only **Type Ib**, removal of the clitoral glans with the prepuce
Type 2	Partial or total removal of the clitoral glans and the labia minora, with or without excision of the labia majora. Sometimes knowns as excision **Type IIa**, removal of the labia minora only **Type IIb**, partial or total removal of the clitoral glans and labia minora **Type IIc**, partial or total removal of the clitoral glans, labia minora and labia majora
Type 3	Narrowing of the vaginal orifice with creation of a covering seal by cutting and appositioning the labia minora and/or the labia majora, with or without excision of the clitoral glans. Sometimes known as infibulation or pharaonic circumcision **Type IIIa**, removal and apposition of the labia minora **Type IIIb**, removal and apposition of the labia majora
Type 4	All other harmful procedures to the female genitalia for non-medical purposes, including Gishiri cuts, pricking, piercing, incising, scraping and cauterisation (and labial elongation)

Adapted from WHO [1]

In 2015, it was estimated that 137 000 women and girls were living with the consequences of FGM in England and Wales [12] and between April 2015 and March 2020, 24 420 health-care attendances by women and girls with FGM were recorded in England [13].

11.2 Classification of FGM Types

Four types of FGM are classified by the WHO (see Table 11.2).

A genital examination should be carried out using a sensitive, culturally competent, trauma-informed approach. The WHO commissioned visual reference guides (see references [14] and [15]), which are a useful resource for health-care professionals who have not come across FGM before.

11.2.1 Classification Challenges

WHO definitions formerly described partial or total removal of the clitoris with Type 1, 2 and 3 FGM. However, during FGM the whole clitoris is never removed as the clitoral body and crux remain deep below the level of the skin layer. Women should be informed that some clitoral tissue always remains intact despite FGM and this explains why women with FGM may still be able to achieve clitoral orgasm.

11.2.1.1 Difficulties Associated with Classification of FGM

- Specific forms of FGM vary from one geographical area to another
- Girls and women rarely know which type they have and may not associate their health problems with the practice as they may have little knowledge of genital anatomy and physiology
- There may be followed by significant variation in the extent of cutting because of poor conditions in which FGM is performed
- FGM does not always leave physical traces. Therefore, a 'normal' genital examination cannot exclude Type 4 FGM/C. Diagnosis should be based on the woman's history not only upon genital assessment
- Type 4 may comprise only a prick or a small scratch and may heal completely leaving no scar or a small scar, which is impossible to detect years later

11.2.1.2 Differential Diagnosis

- Labial adhesion following inflammatory processes or lichen sclerosis can be confused with infibulation
- Small irregularities in the skin of the vulva or clitoris can be a result of congenital variation
- It should be noted that it is not possible to deduce a timeline for an FGM procedure unless it is visualised within a few weeks of being carried out

11.2.2 Some Useful Definitions

Table 11.3 outlines the broad definitions utilised.

Table 11.3 Deinfibulation, reinfibulation and FGM reconstruction

Deinfibulation	Opening the sealed introitus of a woman who has been infibulated to expose the vaginal opening and urinary meatus
Simple deinfibulation	Deinfibulation procedure is carried out under local anaesthetic on the same day in an outpatient or community setting. There is no attempt to expose the clitoral glans and/or prepuce
Complex deinfibulation	Where Type 3 FGM is accompanied by a cyst, fused anterior scar or keloid scar, deinfibulation should be carried out by a suitably trained doctor. This usually requires epidural, spinal or general anaesthesia and is undertaken in theatre as a day case surgery. There may be an attempt to expose clitoral tissue [16]
Reinfibulation	The procedure to narrow the vaginal opening in a woman after she has been deinfibulated (i.e. after childbirth); also known as re-suturing. Commonly carried out in Somalia, Sudan and Saudi Arabia
Reconstruction	This is where skin is grafted to restore original genital appearance. This is currently available in some countries in Europe and Africa and parts of USA.

Table 11.4 Summary of short- and long-term complications

Short-term complications	Long-term complications
Severe pain and injury to genitals	Scarring/keloid formation, Epidermoid cysts/abscesses, Neuroma, Vesicovaginal Fistula
Haemorrhage and haemorrhagic shock	Haematocolpos and dysmenorrhoea
Infection (e.g. tetanus, sepsis)	Dysuria
Urinary retention	Pelvic inflammatory disease/infertility
Trauma to adjacent tissue	Vaginal/urinary/reproductive tract infections
Transmission of blood borne viruses (Hepatitis B, HIV)	Morbidity and mortality during pregnancy and childbirth
Fracture of bones (from being held down)	Psychological and psychosexual problems
Death	Dyspareunia, apareunia, decreased satisfaction

11.3 Health Complications of FGM

Table 11.4 describes some of the common health consequences of FGM.

11.3.1 FGM and Psychological Consequences

Women with FGM are at increased risk of post-traumatic stress disorder, anxiety, depression and low self-esteem [1]. Psychological trauma may be severe with all FGM types. Women report problems such as touch and needle phobia, flashbacks, nightmares and distorted body image, for example 'not feeling whole' [7]. Psychosexual issues include suffering pain during sexual intercourse, lower desire and reduced sexual satisfaction when compared to uncut women [17].

FGM survivors have multiple disadvantages being women who are predominantly from Black, Asian and Minority ethnic communities, and have suffered a serious sexual assault. A high proportion are vulnerable refugee or asylum seekers and are therefore at increased risk of experiencing other forms of intersectional gender-based violence [18], such as forced early marriage, domestic violence, witchcraft/juju, trafficking or enslavement [19]. High cumulative lifetime trauma exposure is also associated with mental health problems [20]. Evidence demonstrates that the disadvantaged often have greater health inequalities and are less likely to be offered, or to access, health care [21].

11.4 Clinical Presentations

At the Sunflower Clinic, an FGM specialist service in London, UK, the most common reasons why FGM survivors present to the clinic are to access either one or a combination of: deinfibulation (often for women who have recently, or are about to, get married); clinical documentation to confirm FGM in support of an asylum application; complex perineal trauma requiring urogynaecology referral; trauma counselling; difficulty in taking cervical smears; and/or diagnosis of FGM type to find out exactly what has been cut [7].

Some of the phrases used by women to describe their FGM symptoms, included: 'severe pain and bleeding during sex'; 'rashes and swelling of genitals'; 'very dry and itchy and burning sensation after intercourse'; 'sore, stuck, itchy labia'; 'can't relax, tense, no lubrication, can't feel anything'; 'unable to have sexual penetration'; 'incontinence'; 'never experienced pleasure'; 'don't feel whole' [7].

11.4.1 FGM Types 1 and 2

Women with FGM types 1 and 2 may suffer long-term psychological and psychosexual complications [7]. Physical problems such as clitoral pain, vulvodynia and epidermoid inclusion cysts (requiring excision and draining under general anaesthetic) are also common.

11.4.2 FGM Type 3

FGM Type 3 is mostly found in the Horn of East Africa in girls between 5–10 years old. It is estimated that eight million women worldwide have suffered Type 3 FGM [1]. It is usually carried out by traditional circumcisers but in urban areas midwives and doctors may be involved. Typically, the child is held down in her own home by members of the family (often female), while without anaesthesia the clitoral glans, prepuce and variable amounts of labia majora or minora are removed (usually cut with a non-sterilised razor blade or knife). The raw edges are then sewn across the midline to produce a barrier of scar tissue, leaving only a small orifice for the passage of urine and menstrual products. Thorns are sometimes used to bring the skin together, especially in remote areas. Traditionally, the legs are bound for several days to restrict movement and promote healing [5]. Women have spoken of their circumciser boasting of the introitus size being equivalent to a grain of rice after the procedure [7].

An intact 'circumcision' may be regarded as a sign of virginity and uncircumcised women are considered unmarriageable. In parts of Somalia, after marriage, it is common for the bridegroom's mother to inspect and confirm 'virginity' and arrange for the traditional circumciser to attend on the wedding night and open up the scar. In other regions of Somalia, the husband is expected to open the introitus himself by forceful intercourse and women have reported subsequent years of excruciating pain [5].

When presenting to a health-care setting, women with Type 3 may say that they have not experienced any health problems from FGM and when asked whether they have difficulty passing urine or painful intercourse, may reply 'it is normal'. However, upon further gentle questioning they may describe their urine as 'dribbling out slowly', sometimes taking 10–20 minutes to empty the bladder. They describe passing blood clots when menstruating and needing to make repeated trips to the family doctor for antibiotics to treat infections [7].

11.4.3 Deinfibulation

Deinfibulation is the opening procedure for a woman with Type 3 FGM. It is sometimes termed a 'reversal', however, it does not replace genital tissue or restore genital anatomy. Deinfibulation is recommended if the introitus is not sufficiently open to permit normal urinary and menstrual flow, comfortable sexual intercourse, to permit cervical smears, sexual health screens and gynaecological surgery such as surgical management of miscarriage or termination of pregnancy, hysteroscopy or endometrial biopsy [22].

Deinfibulation can usually be performed under local anaesthetic as a day case in an outpatient setting. Emla cream can be applied to numb the scar prior to administering Xylocaine 1% (lidocaine 1% with adrenaline). A scissors or a blade is used to incise the scar. Bleeding is usually minimal. Once the urinary meatus has been exposed, the incision may be extended with care into the clitoral region if it appears that the remaining anterior scar is tight and will prevent comfortable sexual intercourse. The raw edges are closed with fine (3/0– 4/0) absorbable sutures such as vicryl rapide, using continuous sutures where possible. The edges should not be left unsutured, as there is a tendency for the scar to re-fuse rendering the Type 3 intact once again after only a few days. Postoperative analgesia such as a long-acting local anaesthetic is injected under the sutured edges (e.g. bupivacaine 0.5%) or Voltarol suppository.

Spinal or general anaesthetic should be offered if the presentation is more complex. For example, if a woman presents with a para-clitoral cyst; is touch or needle phobic; if there is a risk of the deinfibulation procedure triggering psychological flashbacks or distress; or the woman's preference.

Time must be taken to counsel the woman before the procedure of the changes to expect post deinfibulation, such as change to vulval appearance, urinary flow and noise when urinating, appearance and volume of menstrual flow, increased vaginal discharge and what to expect when having sexual intercourse for the first time. It is not uncommon for the clitoral glans to be found present and undamaged during deinfibulation [23].

11.4.4 FGM Type 4

FGM Type 4 includes other unclassified injury to the genital area such as scraping, labial stretching and burning or the introduction of corrosive substances into the vagina. Some of these procedures have serious long-term complications:

> Gynaetresia is recorded in Ibadan, Nigeria. Caustic pessaries are administered by traditional healers to treat amenorrhoea, infertility, fibroids and vaginal discharge. They are also used in an attempt to procure abortion. Of the 148 cases documented at University College Hospital, Ibadan, between 1967 and 1996, 106 required extensive vaginoplasty [24].

Gishiri cuts are incisions into (usually) the anterior vagina by traditional healers to treat a variety of conditions including obstructed labour, infertility, dyspareunia, amenorrhoea, goitre and backache. In one study from Nigeria, '13% of vesico-vaginal fistulae were caused by Gishiri cuts' [25].

11.5 Management of Pregnant Women Presenting to a Maternity Setting

All pregnant women should be asked at booking whether they have been subjected to FGM. If yes, the woman should be referred to an FGM expert (midwife or doctor) preferably in a specialist clinic setting where she can access specialist health advocates and counsellors for holistic support. Appropriate non-judgemental language should be used. Some women may have never spoken of their FGM before so due consideration to this fact should be made. Gentle and sensitive questioning using a trauma-informed, culturally competent approach is necessary. The terms 'cut' or 'circumcision' are usually universally understood. Interpreters should not be a family member, friend or someone with influence in the girl or woman's community as FGM is a very sensitive topic and the woman should be confident that the discussion is confidential. Traditional and local terms for FGM are displayed in a table provided by the UK Department of Health guidance document, FGM Safeguarding and Risk Assessment [26].

11.5.1 Obstetric and Neonatal Risks Associated with FGM

One large prospective study by the WHO investigated both maternal and perinatal outcomes in 28000 women in six African countries. A meta-analysis by Berg et al. reviewed maternal outcomes and included some studies from Western countries (USA and Europe). They reported an increased risk of prolonged labour, postpartum haemorrhage and perineal trauma. The WHO study also found an increased risk of caesarean section and demonstrated an increased need for neonatal resuscitation and risk of stillbirth and early neonatal death [22].

The study concluded that women living with FGM are significantly more likely than those who have not had FGM to have adverse obstetric outcomes [9]. In addition, women with Type 3 will suffer more complications during childbirth than women with other FGM types due to scarring and reduced skin elasticity of the introitus [27].

Screening for HIV, hepatitis B and C should be made available as the use of non-sterile equipment during the original procedure places women with FGM at higher risk of these infections. Clinicians should also be aware that flashbacks may be triggered during vaginal examination or post-partum perineal suturing.

11.5.2 A Holistic Best Practice Consultation Should Include:

(1) Welcoming the woman and encouraging her to voice any pregnancy concerns. The presence of a suitably qualified health advocate who is herself from an FGM practising community is preferable to reassure the woman that she is in a safe environment.

(2) The physical and psychological health consequences of FGM types should be explained in detail using line drawings. FGM Type 1 or clitoroidectomy is sometimes regarded as a less traumatic alternative to other forms of mutilation. Women are reported to sometimes say their FGM was 'just a bleed' or 'just a little cut'. It is important that health-care professionals are clear that no type of FGM is permissible. The infographic from Barnardo's National FGM Centre shown in Figure 11.1 could be a useful resource.

(3) Women (and partners) should be informed that women with any type of FGM are at higher risk of obstetric complications. All primigravida women (and multigravida women if they have not delivered before at that hospital) should be encouraged to consent to a genital assessment to diagnose the FGM type so that a personalised birth plan can be devised. A mirror can be used if the woman wants to be shown exactly what has been cut

(4) A discussion around the law, explaining that FGM is a human rights violation, form of child sexual abuse and that it removes a woman's right to bodily integrity and sexual pleasure should occur. Barnardo's National FGM Centre world prevalence

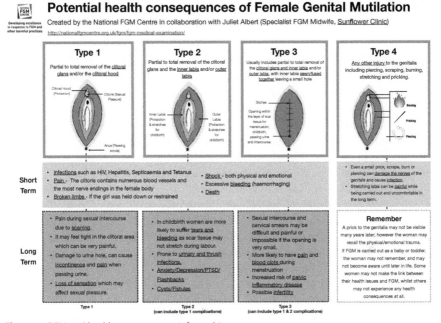

Fig 11.1 FGM and health consequences infographic
Available from: http://nationalfgmcentre.org.uk/wp-content/uploads/2022/03/FGM-and-Health-Consequences-Infographic-2022.pdf

map can be used to discuss the type of FGM, terms used and legal status of FGM in the woman's country of origin.

Recording and Reporting of FGM

(5) A detailed medical history should be taken, documenting any symptoms related to FGM. Questions should include: Who performed the FGM? Did they use pain relief? Were there any complications afterwards? Has FGM caused any health problems, such as difficulty passing urine? Have you ever suffered nightmares or flashbacks?

(6) Referral for psychological assessment and treatment if required

(7) In England, it is mandatory to record prevalence data in accordance with the NHS Digital FGM Enhanced Dataset [28]. This includes age when FGM took place, country where FGM was performed, date of entry to UK (if applicable) and past history of deinfibulation and/or reinfibulation.

(8) An individual risk assessment should be made using an FGM safeguarding assessment tool. An example of such a tool can be found at FGM Professional Guidance (publishing.service.gov.uk)

The woman should be asked: How old were you when you were cut? Where was it carried out? Were other girls cut at the same time, such as siblings or cousins? Who arranged the cut or circumcision and do you know why it was done? Does your family still practise FGM? How does your partner feel about FGM? Does your partner's family believe in practising FGM? Do you have female children or younger siblings who have been cut? An appropriate safeguarding referral should be made if a woman discloses that she has a child under 18 years old who has had FGM or if she knows of a child or unborn child that might be at risk of FGM [22]

11.6 Management of Pregnant Women with Type 3 FGM

It is important to note that pregnancy can occur even with a pinhole opening. Women may also have been reinfibulated after childbirth, therefore multigravida women also require sensitive enquiry during pregnancy.

Antenatal discussion of the benefits of deinfibulation prior to labour should include an explanation that if she has Type 3, she may be more likely to suffer urinary tract or candida infections during pregnancy. There may be a higher risk of difficulty in intrapartum monitoring (including application of fetal scalp electrodes and fetal blood sampling), difficulty in catheterisation during labour, increased risk of prolonged labour and higher incidence of stillbirth, neonatal death, wound infection and retention of lochia [11, 22].

The woman and partner should be counselled to understand that if she has a precipitate delivery, or if she gives birth without a health-care professional/traditional birth attendant present, there is the possibility of fetal asphyxia or anoxia, and/or extensive maternal perineal damage including fistulae.

Simple deinfibulation may be performed either antenatally, in the first stage of labour, at the time of delivery under local anaesthetic or perioperatively after caesarean section [22]. In Africa, women would usually be deinfibulated in the second stage of labour by a traditional birth attendant or midwife.

11.6.1 Antenatal Deinfibulation

Where adequate vaginal assessment in labour is unlikely to be possible, deinfibulation should be recommended in the second trimester, typically at around 20 weeks of gestation. This is to avoid the woman assuming that a spontaneous miscarriage is the result of the operation [22].

There are many advantages of antenatal deinfibulation. For example, an experienced clinician is present, there is no need to rush as the woman is not in labour; the area will be well healed before the onset of labour and therefore, the anterior incision is less likely to extend anteriorly; the woman does not have a baby to look after so can care for the wound site more easily; doing a vaginal examination or inserting a urinary catheter will be more comfortable.

Some women will refuse this, because they fear two episodes of pain, or they may not be identified with Type 3 FGM during pregnancy.

11.6.2 Intrapartum Deinfibulation

Where possible a detailed plan for intrapartum care should be documented and discussed with the woman and her partner. If vaginal examination, intrapartum procedures (e.g. inserting a pessary for induction of labour) and urinary catheterisation are not possible because of the introitus size, then deinfibulation in the first stage of labour is required.

In most maternity units deinfibulation will be delayed until the second stage if possible, as there may be significant blood loss if it is carried out in the first stage of labour.

At delivery, the incision should be made with scissors (rather than a scalpel) just before crowning of the fetal head. Lidocaine should be used. Once the procedure has been performed, the need for episiotomy should be assessed. Medio-lateral episiotomy should only be carried out after an anterior incision is made, as it may not be required. Bilateral episiotomy is never indicated in these cases.

Women should always be informed that reinfibulation is illegal. A woman whose planned deinfibulation was not performed (because of delivery by Caesarean section) should have follow-up in a gynaecology outpatient or FGM clinic so that deinfibulation can be offered before a subsequent pregnancy.

11.7 Safeguarding and Law

FGM is condemned by a number of international treaties and conventions, as well as by national legislation in many countries. For example:

- Article 25 of the Universal Declaration of Human Rights states that 'everyone has the right to a standard of living adequate for health and well-being'
- The UN Convention on the Elimination of All Forms of Discrimination against Women
- The Convention against Torture and Other Cruel, Inhuman, or Degrading Treatment or Punishment
- Convention on the Rights of the Child [8]

In 2018, FGM remained legal in six African countries, Sudan, Somalia, Chad, Mali, Sierra Leone and Liberia. In July 2020, Sudan passed legislation banning the practice across the whole country, however recent unrest has raised concerns that the law may yet go unenforced.

A report by 28 Too Many in 2021 estimates more than 600 000 women and girls in Europe have experienced FGM and a further 130 000 are at risk of FGM. However, prevalence data are sparse, particularly in countries of Eastern Europe.

Some countries have laws to ensure that relevant professionals and institutions are obliged to report FGM cases. In the UK, the first law against FGM was legislated in 1985. In England and Wales, the Serious Crime Act, 2015 introduced new legislation including:

- Mandatory Reporting Duty – all regulated health and social care professionals and teachers are mandated by law to report 'known' cases of FGM in girls under 18 years of age to the police as well as to social care. 'Known' cases are those where a girl herself discloses that she has undergone FGM or where a professional observes evidence on a girl's genitals that she may have been cut [29]
- Failure to Protect Clause – makes it a criminal offence if parents fail to prevent their daughters undergoing FGM by extended family/community members
- FGM Protection Orders – a judge decides how to protect a girl who is at risk of FGM (e.g. by restricting travel outside of the UK until age of 18)
- Enhanced Dataset – it is mandatory for family doctors, mental health trust and hospital foundation trusts to record health service attendances of women and girls identified with FGM

11.8 Conclusion

FGM includes a number of harmful traditional practices, which are a danger to health and an abuse of young women and children. It is important that health professionals are aware of the best management options during pregnancy and childbirth.

Clinical Governance Issues

- FGM is a form of child sexual abuse and a human rights violation
- Women should always be treated sensitively using a trauma-informed and culturally safe approach
- Consultation with a woman (and partner) with FGM is an opportunity to explain the health consequences of FGM and to help prevent the continuation of the practice
- FGM is usually performed by traditional cutters but rates of medicalised cutting are increasing
- Pregnant women and their partners should be informed that they are at higher risk of adverse obstetric outcomes because of FGM
- Deinfibulation should be performed to reduce the complications of Type 3 FGM
- Women with Type 3 FGM should be informed of the benefits of antenatal deinfibulation preferably under local anaesthetic in the second trimester

References

1   WHO. *Female Genital Mutilation. Key Facts.* [Internet]. (2021), 1–5. www.who.int/en/news-room/fact-sheets/detail/female-genital-mutilation

2   WHO. *Eliminating Female Genital Mutilation: An Interagency Statement UNAIDS, UNDP, UNECA, UNESCO, UNFPA, UNHCHR, UNHCR, UNICEF, UNIFEM, WHO.* (2008). http://apps.who.int/iris/bitstream/handle/10665/43839/9789241596442_eng.pdf.;jsessionid=996E4B151551E5B1C8D31AFC670234BE?sequence=1

3   United Nations. *Transforming Our World: The 2030 Agenda for Sustainable Development.* (2015). https://sustainabledevelopment.un.org/content/documents/21252030

4   U. Elchalal, B. Ben-Ami, R. Gillis and A. Brzezinski. Ritualistic female genital mutilation. *Obstetrical & Gynecologial Survey*, **52** (1997), 643–51.

5   H. Gordon. Female genital mutilation. In A. H. Sultan, R. Thakar and D. E. Fenner, eds., *Perineal and Anal Sphincter Trauma.* (London: Springer, 2009). https://doi.org/10.1007/978-1-84628-503-5_7

6   United Nations Children's Fund. *Female Genital Mutilation: A New Generation Calls for Ending an Old Practice.* (New York: UNICEF, 2020).

7   J. Albert and M. Wells. The Acton Model: Support for women with female genital mutilation. *British Journal of Midwifery* [Internet], **28** (2020), 697–708. www.magonlinelibrary.com/doi/10.12968/bjom.2020.28.10.697

8   UNICEF. *Female Genital Mutilation* [Internet]. (2021). https://data.unicef.org/topic/child-protection/female-genital-mutilation/

9   UNICEF. *Female Genital Mutilation/Cutting: A Global Concern* [Internet]. (2016). www.who.int/en/news-room/fact-sheets/detail/female-genital-mutilation

10   Population Council. *Evidence to End FGM/C: Research to Help Girls and Women Thrive* [Internet]. (2020). file:///C:/Users/44773/Documents/research articles/2020RH_FGMC_ReflectionsFiveYears.pdf

11   WHO. *Care of Women and Girls Living with Female Genital Mutilation: A Clinical Handbook.* [Internet]. (2018). file:///C:/Users/44773/Downloads/9789241513913-eng.pdf

12   A. J. Macfarlane and E. Dorkenoo. Estimating the numbers of women and

girls with female genital mutilation in England and Wales. *Journal of Epidemiology an Community Health* [Internet], **69** (2015). https://openaccess.city.ac.uk/id/eprint/12382

13 S. Karlsen, J. Howard, N. Carver, M. Mogilnicka and C. Pantazis. Available evidence suggests that prevalence and risk of female genital cutting/mutilation in the UK is much lower than widely presumed – policies based on exaggerated estimates are harmful to girls and women from affected communities. *International Journal of Impotence Research* [Internet], (2022). www.nature.com/articles/s41443-021-00526-4

14 J. Abdulcadir, L. Catania, M. J. Hindin, et al. Female genital mutilation: A visual reference and learning tool for health care professionals. *Obstetrics & Gynecology* [Internet], **128** (2016), 958–63. www.ncbi.nlm.nih.gov/pubmed/27741194

15 J. Abdulcadir, S. Marras, L. Catania, O. Abdulcadir and P. Petignat. Defibulation: A visual reference and learning tool. *Journal of Sexual Medicine* [Internet], **15** (2018), 601–11. https://doi.org/10.1016/j.jsxm.2018.01.010

16 J. Abdulcadir, M. Rodriguez and L. Say. Research gaps in the care of women with female genital mutilation: An analysis. *BJOG: An International Journal of Obstetrics and Gynaecology* [Internet], **122** (2015), 294–303. http://doi.wiley.com/10.1111/1471-0528.13217

17 R. C. Berg, S. Taraldsen, M. A. Said, I. K. Sørbye and S. Vangen. Reasons for and experiences with surgical interventions for female genital mutilation/cutting (FGM/C): A systematic review. *Journal of Sexual Medicine* [Internet], **14** (2017), 977–90. https://linkinghub.elsevier.com/retrieve/pii/S1743609517312663

18 GOV.UK. *Multi-Agency Statutory Guidance on Female Genital Mutilation* [Internet]. (2016). https://assets.publishing.service.gov.uk/government/uploads/system/uploads/attachment_data/file/800306/6-1914-HO-Multi_Agency_Statutory_Guidance.pdf

19 WHO. *WHO Guidelines on the Management of Health Complications From Female Genital Mutilation* [Internet]. (2016). www.who.int/reproductivehealth/topics/fgm/management-health-complications-fgm/en/

20 J. Ormrod. The experience of NHS care for women living with female genital mutilation. *British Journal of Nursing,* **28** (2019), 628–33.

21 H. Watson, D. Harrop, E. Walton, A. Young and H. Soltani. A systematic review of ethnic minority women's experiences of perinatal mental health conditions and services in Europe. *PLoS One* [Internet], **14** (2019), e0210587. https://dx.plos.org/10.1371/journal.pone.0210587

22 Royal College of Obstetricians and Gynaecologists. *Female Genital Mutilation and its Management. RCOG Green-top Guideline No. 53* [Internet]. (2015). www.rcog.org.uk/globalassets/documents/guidelines/gtg-53-fgm.pdf

23 H. Gordon. H. Comerasamy and N. H. Morris. Female genital mutilation: Experience in a West London clinic. *Journal of Obstetrics and Gynaecology,* **27** (2007),416–19.

24 O. Arowojolu, M. A. Okunlola, A. O. Adekunle and A.O. Ilesanmi. Three decades of acquired gynaetresia in Ibadan: Clinical presentation and management. *Journal of Obstetrics and Gynaecology (Lahore)* [Internet], **21** (2001), 375–8. www.tandfonline.com/doi/full/10.1080/01443610120059923

25 F. Tahzib. Epidemiological determinants of vesicovaginal fistulas. *British Journal of Obstetrics and Gynaecology,* **90** (1983), 387–91.

26 E. Banks, O. Meirik, T. Farley, O. Akande and H. AM. Bathija. Female genital mutilation and obstetric outcome: WHO collaborative prospective study in six

African countries. *Lancet* [Internet], **367** (2006), 1835–41. https://linkinghub .elsevier.com/retrieve/pii/ S0140673606688053

27 Department of Health. *FGM Safeguarding and Risk Assessment: Quick Guide for Health Professionals*. [Internet]. (2017). https://assets.publishing.service .gov.uk/government/uploads/system/ uploads/attachment_data/file/585083/ FGM_safeguarding_and_risk_assessment .pdf

28 NHS Digital. *Female Genital Mutilation Datasets* [Internet]. (2020). https://digital .nhs.uk/data-and-information/clinical-audits-and-registries/female-genital-mutilation-datasets

29 Department of Health. *Female Genital Mutilation Risk and Safeguarding; Guidance for Professionals*. (FGM Prevention Programme, London, 2016), available at Female Genital Mutilation Risk and Safeguarding (publishing.service .gov.uk).

Chapter 12

Ovarian and Cervical Malignancy in Pregnancy

Helen Bolton

12.1 Background

Cancer during pregnancy is rare, affecting approximately 1 in 1,000 pregnancies [1]. Although rare, most obstetricians will at times be responsible for women who have a history of cancer, or present with symptoms or signs of possible malignancy during pregnancy, or even encounter a new diagnosis during a current pregnancy. Pregnancy itself does not predispose to cancer, but there may be delays in diagnosis due to symptoms being falsely attributed to physiological symptoms related to pregnancy.

There is often limited, if any, data to direct evidence-based management of women affected by gynaecological cancer in pregnancy. The European Society for Medical Oncology (ESMO) has published helpful guidelines on management of these women, based on a combination of the current evidence available and international expert consensus [2].

12.2 General Principles of Managing Cancer in Pregnancy

The management of any cancer always requires a multidisciplinary team (MDT) approach, but when the patient is pregnant the MDT will also need to involve the patient's obstetrician and often the neonatal team. Many obstetricians do not manage gynaecological malignancies routinely, however when cancer occurs during pregnancy, they will become a key member of the MDT. Similarly, many oncologists have limited experience in managing pregnant women and will need to work collaboratively with the patient's obstetric team to ensure the best overall outcome from her cancer and her pregnancy.

Treatment decisions must always consider both maternal and fetal concerns, taking into consideration the urgency of treatment, prognosis and maternal views. Whenever possible, women should receive standard treatment of their cancer, while minimising the risks of prematurity or pregnancy loss. All efforts should be made to continue the pregnancy wherever safe and feasible.

Women with cancer should be cared for in a high-risk obstetric setting, in collaboration with obstetricians, cancer specialists and neonatal expertise. Accurate assessment of gestational age is essential for appropriate timing of intervention. The neonatal team should be aware of the treatment during pregnancy, to ensure appropriate paediatric assessment and follow-up. Malignancy is an additional risk factor for venous thromboembolism and the indication for thromboprophylaxis should be reviewed regularly throughout pregnancy and the post-partum period. Breastfeeding is usually acceptable unless chemotherapy has been given within the last three weeks or if other oncological drugs are being taken. Women and their families should be offered access to psychological support wherever possible.

Imaging during pregnancy should be adapted to avoid exposure to any ionising radiation, to protect the fetus. This contrasts with women who are not pregnant, where CT and PET-CT are frequently indicated. MRI is often a suitable alternative to CT in pregnancy. MRI interpretation may be more challenging due to fetal movement and the presence of dilated pelvic veins

Surgery can usually be carried out safely in pregnancy and is often the primary treatment modality for many cancers. Adapting the procedure or postponing surgery in selected cases may be necessary. The optimal timing for any surgery during pregnancy is early second trimester, with a lower risk of miscarriage than the first trimester, while the size of the uterus should still enable adequate pelvic access. Laparoscopy may be feasible with an experienced surgical team, although standard treatment for gynaecological cancers often requires laparotomy. Beyond 22 weeks, standard pelvic surgery may not be possible due to limited pelvic access. Surgery should be carried out in collaboration with the obstetric team, with an anaesthetic and theatre team experienced in undertaking obstetric anaesthesia. From around 20 weeks, women should be placed in the left lateral tilt position, although this may become necessary at an earlier gestation for women with large ovarian masses.

Chemotherapy can be given in pregnancy but is contraindicated in the first trimester due to the potential teratogenic effects. It should be avoided in the last few weeks prior to delivery, to allow maternal and fetal bone marrow suppression time to recover. Most chemotherapy agents cross the placenta. Breastfeeding is contraindicated during chemotherapy. Newer non-cytotoxic systemic cancer treatments such as bevacizumab, immune checkpoint inhibitors and poly ADP ribose polymerase (PARP) inhibitors should be avoided throughout pregnancy and while breastfeeding due to limited safety data.

Pelvic radiotherapy is absolutely contraindicated in pregnancy. Neoadjuvant chemotherapy (NACT) can be considered in some cases as an alternative non-standard approach to control disease if deferring treatment, termination of pregnancy or elective preterm delivery are not feasible or agreeable options.

12.3 Cervical Cancer

12.3.1 Pre-Malignant Cervical Conditions

In England, the National Health Service Cervical Screening Programme invites women between the ages of 24.5–64 years to participate in a national screening programme [3]. During pregnancy, it is usual to delay a routine screening test until after delivery. Cervical cytology in pregnancy may cause unnecessary concern due to the presence of decidual cells which can be mistaken for dyskaryosis.

Similarly, it is safe and usually advisable to defer monitoring of low-grade abnormalities or screening samples after treatment ('test of cure') until after delivery [4]. However, colposcopy may be indicated during pregnancy in cases of high-grade pre-invasive disease.

Colposcopy in pregnancy is safe with no impact on the pregnancy, although it is good practice to keep the obstetrician updated. However colposcopy will be technically challenging due to physiological changes in the cervix, often appearing suspicious to an inexperienced practitioner. It should only be carried out by an appropriately qualified clinician, if indicated [3]. In contrast to women who are not pregnant, the primary aim of colposcopy during pregnancy is solely to identify cancer, avoiding biopsy or treatment until after delivery, where the colposcopist judges it is safe to do so. Excision or biopsy should be avoided but must be carried out with appropriate care if cancer is suspected. Women with high-grade disease in early pregnancy should be reviewed again in the late second trimester, and further follow-up in pregnancy arranged at the clinician's discretion.

Post-partum health-care systems must ensure that women are not lost to screening or follow-up as a consequence of deferral during pregnancy. Maternity services should use the opportunity of public health promotion to educate and encourage women to attend for routine screening from three months post-partum, where appropriate.

12.3.2 Previous History of Cervical Malignancy

Women with a history of early-stage cervical cancer may have had fertility-sparing treatment, such as excision of the transformation zone or trachelectomy. Those with more advanced disease require treatment that invariably results in loss of fertility.

Treatment for very early-stage (1A) disease includes large loop excision of the transformation zone (LLETZ) or cone biopsy [5]. These women may be at higher risk of mid-trimester pregnancy loss and preterm birth. The risk increases for women who have had deeper excisions (>10 mm) or more than one treatment [6]; both being risk factors more likely in women undergoing LLETZ for cancer, rather than pre-invasive disease alone.

For early, low volume stage IB cervical cancers, women may have been treated by trachelectomy (simple or radical); a technique specifically used for women wishing to have a future pregnancy. Trachelectomy involves removal of the cervix (simple trachelectomy) together with the surrounding parametrium and upper vagina (radical trachelectomy), with anastomosis of the uterine isthmus or proximal cervix to the vagina. Most women have a non-absorbable cervical cerclage suture placed at the uterine isthmus during the procedure, with the intention of providing a mechanical barrier. Potential reproductive issues affecting women with a history of trachelectomy include lower spontaneous conception rates, increased risk of first and second trimester miscarriage, together with preterm birth. First trimester miscarriage rates are similar to the general population. Second trimester loss is estimated at around 7%, and usually associated with infection and preterm, premature rupture of the membranes (PPROM), with preterm delivery rates ranging between 20–45% [7].

12.3.2.1 Antepartum Management
Women with a history of simple excisional treatment such as LLETZ

Ideally women should have been counselled about the potential risks of mid-trimester loss and preterm birth at the time of their treatment, however the routine antenatal history should always include a specific enquiry about previous history of cervical treatment in case this is not volunteered. It is particularly helpful for the obstetrician to be aware of the depth and number of treatments to help evaluate the potential increase in risk to the pregnancy.

For those pregnancies judged to be at high risk, such as those women with deep and/or repeated LLETZ treatments, a second trimester transvaginal ultrasound scan may be helpful to identify a short cervix and consideration of ultrasound-indicated cervical cerclage.

Women with a history of trachelectomy

Evidence-based guidance on the management of pregnancies with a previous history of trachelectomy are limited. Several recent review articles have been published summarising the evidence available, and sharing expert approach and guidance based on this evidence and experience [8, 9].

If first trimester miscarriage occurs, a medical management approach is favoured which should avoid disrupting the cerclage. If surgical evacuation is required, this should be carried out by a senior clinician, often with ultrasound guidance to minimise the risk of uterine perforation. Locating the neo-cervical os can difficult.

The management of second trimester miscarriage and infection is especially challenging as the cervical cerclage may need to be removed. This can be replaced in a subsequent pregnancy. An abdominal cerclage may be required if the cervix is too short.

The focus in pregnancy should be on managing the significant risk of preterm delivery. Trachelectomy is likely to result in subsequent compromise of the mechanical, biochemical and immunological barriers of the cervix, consequently resulting in a higher risk of ascending infection with increased risk of second trimester miscarriage, chorioamnionitis, premature rupture of the membranes and preterm labour. Due to a lack of data in this population group, studies on women with cervical insufficiency are usually extrapolated to guide management. A variety of interventions have been proposed to manage these pregnancies including screening and treatment of asymptomatic bacteriuria, fetal fibronectin testing and serial cervical ultrasound assessment to assess for length and progressive shortening [8, 9]. An additional suture is not usually an option if cervical shortening or dilatation occurs, because of insufficient cervical length resulting from the trachelectomy. Vaginal progesterone supplementation may be considered from 12 weeks. Avoiding strenuous activity, sexual activity and digital vaginal examinations have also been recommended, although there is no evidence to support these measures in the absence of complications. Prophylactic steroids should be given from 24 weeks if delivery is imminent or there are signs of preterm labour. If PPROM occurs, antibiotics and steroids should be administered with a view to delivery as per standard guidelines.

12.3.2.2 Intrapartum Management
Women with a history of simple excisional treatment such as LLETZ

Patients with a previous history of simple excisional treatment have no specific contra-indications to vaginal birth. Cervical stenosis is an uncommon consequence of treatment, and may result in labour dystocia, requiring emergency Caesarean delivery.

Women with a history of trachelectomy

There is consensus that women with a history of trachelectomy should avoid labour and be advised to deliver by Caesarean section [8, 9]. Attempts at spontaneous birth may be complicated by severe haemorrhage due to lateral cervical tears or uterine rupture. Delivery is usually timed at around 37 weeks to avoid spontaneous labour, with a low threshold for earlier delivery in the presence of PPROM or suspected labour, which can be difficult to diagnose in these patients. Caesarean delivery may be complicated by distorted anatomy, including an absent lower segment. This increases the risk of extension of a low transverse excision directly into the uterine arteries with resulting major haemorrhage. Although this can be avoided by carrying out a classical midline uterine incision, consideration should be given to the feasibility and safety of a transverse incision to minimise the potential risks to future pregnancies, if relevant. These issues should be anticipated in advance, with an experienced obstetrician performing the Caesarean, and adequate preparation for major haemorrhage.

12.3.2.3 Post-Partum Management

All women should be provided with adequate post-natal support, including encouragement to continue to engage with their cancer follow-up pathway, if relevant.

12.3.3 Cervical Cancer in Pregnancy

Cervical cancer is the most common gynaecological malignancy diagnosed during pregnancy, although it remains rare with an incidence estimated between 0.1–12 per 10,000 pregnancies. Symptoms of cervical cancer may mimic those of pregnancy, leading to delays in diagnosis. Obstetricians must maintain a high index of suspicion, with a low threshold for examination and referral for diagnostics. Clear referral pathways should be in place for obstetricians to access urgent assessment for suspected cervical cancer by an experienced gynaecologist or colposcopist.

Once the diagnosis is confirmed, the subsequent management of cervical cancer and the pregnancy is complex, and will depend upon the stage of cancer, gestation of the pregnancy, together with the woman's individual wishes.

12.3.3.1 Symptoms and Diagnosis

Cervical cancer may be diagnosed in pregnancy following an abnormal screening test or as a result of investigations undertaken due to symptoms. Symptoms are related to the stage of disease, and do not differ between pregnant and non-pregnant women. Painless spontaneous vaginal bleeding, post-coital bleeding and vaginal discharge are all presenting symptoms of local cervical cancer. As cancer progresses, pelvic and back pain, urinary and bowel symptoms develop as signs of locally advanced disease. These symptoms are common in pregnancy; hence, the potential risk of delayed diagnosis due to incorrect attribution. Presentation with distant metastatic disease is rare.

12.3.3.2 Staging of Cervical Cancer in Pregnancy

Once a diagnosis of cervical cancer has been established, clinical examination and imaging investigations are required to stage the cancer and direct subsequent management. The International Federation of Gynaecology and Obstetrics (2018) staging system is currently used and applicable in pregnancy [10]. Pelvic MRI is the first line imaging modality for staging of cervical cancer and is safe in pregnancy. Outside of pregnancy, CT or PET-CT is used to evaluate for distant metastases. However, during pregnancy the need for information that guides maternal management must be balanced with the requirement to minimise the exposure of the fetus to ionising radiation. CT or chest X-ray (CXR), with fetal shielding, may be carried out to evaluate for chest metastases in higher risk cases. Radiologists should be directly involved in imaging planning.

Histologically proven regional lymph node involvement is indicative of advanced stage disease (stage IIIC or above), irrespective of the extent of local disease or macroscopically normal lymph nodes on imaging. Women who are less than around 22 weeks gestation, with imaging and examination findings suggestive of stage IA2 to IB2 disease, may benefit from assessment with surgical pelvic lymphadenectomy (if technically feasible), if they are considering delaying their treatment to allow time for fetal maturation. The role of staging lymphadenectomy should be carefully considered in the cancer MDT meeting, taking into account the woman's wishes. Although sentinel lymph node biopsy is sometimes used in staging, the role in pregnancy remains unclear. Until further trials are carried out to assess safety and accuracy, sentinel lymph node biopsy (SLNB) should not be performed in pregnancy outside of trials [5].

12.3.3.3 Principles of Management of Cervical Cancer in Pregnancy

The management of cervical cancer during pregnancy is challenging, and will depend on the gestational age at the time of diagnosis, the stage of the cancer and the woman's underlying wishes after careful counselling. High-risk rare histological subtypes, such as clear cell and small cell endocrine tumours may necessitate a less conservative approach for the best possible treatment outcome.

Women should be made aware of the option of termination of pregnancy in early pregnancy, and the potential implications of premature delivery if needed in later gestations. Women who opt for non-standard treatment due to their pregnancy should be advised that their cancer outcomes may be less certain or optimal than with standard treatment.

Treatment without delay is usually recommended for cervical cancer, regardless of gestation, if there are confirmed lymph node metastases, evidence of disease progression during the pregnancy or if the patient chooses to discontinue the pregnancy [2].

Termination of pregnancy is an option for women in early pregnancy, subject to local legal statutes. For early-stage disease, treated surgically, it is usually recommended that surgery is carried out with the embryo or fetus *in situ*. For patients requiring chemoradiation, it is preferable to complete termination prior to treatment where possible.

Gestational age at diagnosis has a significant impact on management approach. Prior to viability treatment, approaches generally include termination of pregnancy with a view to proceeding with standard treatment, delaying standard treatment until after delivery or NACT to help treat and control the disease, followed by standard treatment after delivery. The management of patients presenting at a more advanced gestational age is focused on fetal maturation, with the option of delayed standard treatment or NACT.

Chemotherapy during pregnancy may be considered prior to definitive treatment, or in a palliative setting for advanced, incurable disease. NACT is the use of chemotherapy prior to definitive treatment. It is not currently used as a standard treatment approach for cervical cancer, although it utilised more often during pregnancy to allow time for fetal maturation [11]. Chemotherapy should be avoided in the first trimester, due to the significant risk of major congenital malformations. Subsequent use of chemotherapy has not shown any evidence of major harm, although data are limited [12].

Surveillance during pregnancy should include regular obstetric assessment by a maternal–fetal medicine specialist. Fetal growth and well-being should be monitored, together with planned oncological surveillance while pregnancy continues. Clinical examination and MRI surveillance can be used to assess for disease progression if standard treatment is being delayed or to assess the response to NACT. Disease progression necessitates an immediate change to standard treatment.

Timing of delivery requires a collaborative obstetric, neonatal and oncological approach. When a decision has been made to adapt the cancer treatment to optimise pregnancy outcome, the aim should be to ensure fetal maturation, avoiding significant risks of iatrogenic prematurity while balancing the best interests of the mother's oncological outcome. Delivery between 34–36 weeks usually strikes the optimal balance, although earlier delivery may be necessary and timing should always be individualised. It may be helpful to involve the neonatal team in discussions with the mother. If NACT has been received, delivery should be timed wherever possible to allow a three-week window following chemotherapy, to minimise the potential impact of bone marrow suppression and risk of infection, on both the mother and her baby.

Mode of delivery should be by Caesarean section in all but the very earliest stages of cervical cancer, with vaginal delivery avoided in the presence of visible tumour [5]. Maternal cancer outcomes are compromised with vaginal delivery.

Breastfeeding is contraindicated during chemotherapy as it crosses into the breast milk, and may cause neonatal leucopoenia and increased risk of sepsis. Women should be warned of this in advance and offered appropriate support. An interval of 14 days from the last chemotherapy session is usually required to ensure clearance from breast milk.

12.3.3.4 Definitive Treatment

Stage IA1 disease is usually diagnosed after excisional treatment and is unlikely to be diagnosed during pregnancy unless carried out as a diagnostic biopsy. The risk of lymph node metastases in stage IA1 is usually less than 1% with no need for further lymph node assessment. In most cases, this should have no significant impact on subsequent pregnancy management, and these patients can be managed as those with a history of simple excisional treatment.

The standard treatment of stages IA2 to IB2 cervical cancer is surgery with radical hysterectomy, bilateral salpingectomy, with bilateral pelvic lymphadenectomy. Pelvic lymphadenectomy for staging may be carried out in early pregnancy, but not in the third trimester [2]. Antenatal trachelectomy is no longer recommended during pregnancy due to evidence showing high rates of surgical and obstetric complications, including haemorrhage and poor fetal outcomes [5].

Women with stage IB3 and above are usually treated with radical chemoradiation after Caesarean delivery or termination of pregnancy. Definitive treatment plans should be reconsidered at MDT level to evaluate treatment response or progression during pregnancy, which may require a different approach.

Consideration should be given to ovarian transposition and bilateral salpingectomy at the time of Caesarean section if definitive surgical treatment is being carried out, or if there are plans for chemoradiation. Ovarian transposition aims to conserve ovarian function from the effects of pelvic radiotherapy; thus, reducing the risk of treatment-induced premature ovarian failure.

12.4 Ovarian Cancer

12.4.1 Previous History of Ovarian Malignancy

Unlike cervical cancer, women with a previous history of ovarian cancer are at less risk of subsequent pregnancy complications. All women with a previous history of malignancy should be reviewed by their obstetrician and a detailed history of their cancer and its previous treatment obtained. If women are still undergoing follow-up after treatment, the obstetric team should liaise with the woman's specialist to discuss the pregnancy and any adaptations to the follow-up plan in the context of her pregnancy. Routine CT imaging and CA-125 monitoring may need to be deferred during pregnancy. If there is clinical suspicion of recurrence during pregnancy, an MRI scan can be performed. Maintenance drugs such as PARP inhibitors should be stopped, ideally prior to pregnancy and after discussion with the oncology team.

12.4.2 Adnexal Mass Presenting in Pregnancy

The use of routine ultrasound for all women during the first and second trimesters of pregnancy means that the coincidental finding of asymptomatic adnexal masses is a common scenario. Only a very small minority are malignant [13], however it is important that these abnormalities are carefully evaluated to ensure appropriate and timely management. Definitive diagnosis can only occur following resection and histological assessment, although surgery during pregnancy should be reserved for cases where malignancy is suspected, or if the cyst is a potential risk to the pregnancy due to mass effects or an acute cyst event such as torsion.

Adequate imaging is required to help evaluate the likelihood of malignancy. Ultrasound imaging is used first line to evaluate the adnexal mass, with various scoring systems published. Complex cysts identified during routine screening may benefit from a second opinion from a clinician experienced in adnexal scanning. MRI may be informative if the adnexal lesion is difficult to evaluate on ultrasound scan, or if there are concerning features that may benefit from a more detailed assessment of morphology. CT should be avoided during pregnancy and is rarely necessary except in exceptional circumstances.

Tumour markers are not routinely helpful when assessed during pregnancy, as they can be difficult to interpret due to physiological elevation and fluctuation during gestation.

Management during pregnancy will depend on the likelihood of malignancy on imaging, or if the adnexal mass is large and compromising the pregnancy through mass effects or ovarian torsion. Smaller benign lesions should be managed conservatively in pregnancy, but with clear plans in place, agreed with the mother in advance, should she require Caesarean delivery. Where malignancy is suspected, surgery is usually recommended after timely review by the cancer MDT.

12.4.3 Suspected Borderline Ovarian Tumours in Pregnancy

Borderline epithelial ovarian tumours are non-invasive epithelial tumours that can sometimes be associated with non-invasive peritoneal implants and spread. They exhibit characteristics on the spectrum between benign cysts and invasive cancer, although they are not considered to be malignant. They are more common in younger women and hence, may be encountered in pregnancy. Borderline ovarian cysts typically exhibit internal papillary projections on ultrasound or MRI, although the diagnosis is only confirmed by histological evaluation following removal of the ovary or ovarian cyst. In general, these tumours have a good prognosis and it is reasonable to manage most cases conservatively during pregnancy with a view to surgical treatment in the post-partum period [2]. All suspected borderline tumours must be reviewed by the cancer MDT. The MDT should provide recommendations on the timing of treatment in addition to plans for any monitoring and surgical treatment approaches. It is helpful for the woman and her obstetric team to have a clearly documented plan supporting deferring treatment until after delivery, if appropriate. In younger women, borderline tumours are often treated conservatively by ovarian cystectomy to preserve ovarian function and fertility, provided there is sufficient underlying normal ovarian tissue to make this approach feasible. Ovarian tissue can often be evaluated on review of the MRI. Ideally, the woman should be seen by the specialist gynaecology team during pregnancy to discuss the findings and agree the treatment approach prior to delivery. A plan should be made in collaboration with the obstetric team regarding surgical treatment should the woman require either an elective or emergency Caesarean section. Provided expertise is available, the cyst can be treated at the time of Caesarean, thus avoiding the need for further surgery post-partum.

Surgical treatment may be required during pregnancy if the cyst is large, symptomatic, or if there are features more concerning for malignancy or significant peritoneal spread.

12.4.4 Suspected Ovarian Malignancy in Pregnancy

Management of suspected ovarian tumours in pregnancy should be guided by the specialist cancer MDT, considering the likelihood of malignancy, the type of tumour suspected and the gestation of pregnancy. Most ovarian tumours in pregnancy present at stage 1, confined to the ovary. As with any suspected cancer in pregnancy, management approaches should aim to adhere to 'standard care' where possible, with alterations in management carefully individualised to balance the maternal needs for treatment of her cancer, against the potential harm to the fetus from treatment, including risks of surgery, radiation exposure, chemotherapy and prematurity.

Malignant tumours affecting pregnant women include epithelial ovarian cancers, germ cell tumours or rarer malignancies such as sex cord stromal tumours and metastatic Krukenberg tumours.

Germ cell tumours are a rare subtype of ovarian malignancy, but more common in younger women, especially below the age of thirty. They are derived from the primordial germ cells of the ovary. In contrast to epithelial ovarian tumours, they often grow rapidly and are typically characterised by pelvic pain as a result of capsular distension. They are usually unilateral and have a typical complex, solid appearance on ultrasound and MRI. Most will present as stage I disease. Standard treatment of stage I disease is for a fertility-sparing approach with laparotomy, unilateral salpingo-oophorectomy and peritoneal staging (washings for cytology, peritoneal biopsies, omentectomy). Post-operative chemotherapy may be indicated in high-risk cases.

Invasive epithelial tumours comprise the most common group of ovarian tumours overall but are less common in pregnancy as they typically affect older women. They may be classified as high or low grade. Standard treatment for suspected invasive epithelial ovarian tumours is laparotomy and full surgical staging, even in suspected stage I disease. For women who have completed their family, this usually includes hysterectomy and bilateral adnexectomy. Standard treatment approaches for patients with metastatic peritoneal disease are highly individualised but generally include a combination of chemotherapy and surgery.

Surgery for suspected ovarian malignancy or tumours in pregnancy should be carried out after the first trimester, if possible, to minimise the risk of miscarriage, and ideally early in the second trimester where the size of the uterus is still small to allow access. Patients with very large ovarian masses or suspected germ cell tumours may require surgery earlier in the pregnancy, due to the potential harms caused by delay. Presentation during the third trimester is rare, as the majority of abnormalities will have been identified on screening. In these cases, the oncology and obstetric teams should consider timing of delivery, balancing the risks of fetal immaturity against the risks of surgery during pregnancy or treatment delay until post-partum. In most situations where ovarian malignancy is suspected, an open (laparotomy) approach is recommended to allow full evaluation of the intra-abdominal cavity, and to minimise the risk of spillage of tumour cells from the ovary on manipulation of the mass. If ovarian malignancy is suspected and confined to a single ovary, a uterine preserving approach of unilateral salpingo-oophorectomy, peritoneal washings and omental biopsies may be carried out, with the caveat that further formal staging surgery or treatment may be required after pregnancy.

Treatment for suspected advanced stage ovarian cancer in pregnancy requires a careful assessment of the likely underlying pathology (particularly distinguishing between germ cell and epithelial ovarian cancers), and usually a combination of surgery and chemotherapy. NACT may be given in the second or third trimester (after confirmation of the tumour subtype with a biopsy), with a view to offering cytoreductive surgery following delivery. Women with advanced epithelial cancer presenting in the first trimester may consider termination of pregnancy.

Clinical Governance Issues

- Pregnancy in women with a past or current history of cervical or ovarian tumours should be considered as high risk and managed using a collaborative approach with the obstetric and oncology teams
- Women who have had treatment to the cervix for cervical intra-epithelial neoplasia (CIN) or cervical cancer should be informed of the potential impact on subsequent pregnancy and encouraged to advise their obstetric team early in the pregnancy
- Routine antenatal booking assessments should always include an enquiry about past history of cancer or pre-cancer treatment
- Women with a previous history of cervical cancer treatment are usually at higher risk of preterm delivery
- Clinicians should be vigilant to symptoms of cancer presenting during pregnancy and investigate where appropriate
- Women with an adnexal mass that may require surgery should have a clear plan agreed antenatally, including the approach to surgery should she require Caesarean delivery

- Women presenting with cancer in pregnancy should be considered for 'standard of care' cancer treatment wherever possible, accepting that alterations will be necessary and justified to balance the needs of the mother with those of the fetus
- Ionising radiation procedures should be avoided if possible, and only carried out after extensive discussion about its clinical relevance in individual cases, with appropriate precautions
- A multidisciplinary approach including the cancer MDT, obstetricians and neonatal team is essential, and must consider maternal wishes

References

1 P. Morice, C. Uzan, S. Gouy, C. Verschraegen and C. Haie-Meder. Gynaecological cancers in pregnancy. *Lancet*, **379** (2012), 558–69.

2 F. Amant, P. Berveiller, I. A. Boere, et al. Gynecologic cancers in pregnancy: Guidelines based on a third international consensus meeting. *Annals of Oncology*, **30** (2019), 1601–12.

3 NHS England Guidance. *Cervical Screening: Programme and Colposcopy Management*. (Public Health England, 2021). www.gov.uk/government/publications/cervical-screening-programme-and-colposcopy-management

4 L. S. Massad, M. H. Einstein, W. K. Huh, et al. 2012 updated consensus guidelines for the management of abnormal cervical cancer screening tests and cancer precursors. *Obstetrics & Gynecology*, **121** (2013), 829–46.

5 N. Reed, J. Balega, T. Barwick, et al. British Gynaecological Cancer Society (BGCS) cervical cancer guidelines: Recommendations for practice. *European Journal of Obstetrics & Gynecology and Reproductive Biology*, **256** (2021), 433–65.

6 M. Kyrgiou, A. Athanasiou, I. E. J. Kalliala, et al. Obstetric outcomes after conservative treatment for cervical intraepithelial lesions and early invasive disease. *Cochrane Database of Systematic Reviews*, **11** (2017), CD012847.

7 E. Bentivegna, A. Maulard, P. Pautier, et al. Fertility results and pregnancy outcomes after conservative treatment of cervical cancer: A systematic review of the literature. *Fertility and Sterility*, **106** (2016), 1195–1211.

8 P. Simjak, D. Cibula, A. Pařízek and J. Sláma. Management of pregnancy after fertility-sparing surgery for cervical cancer. *Acta Obstetrics at Gynecologica Scandinavica*, **99** (2020), 830–8.

9 Y. Kasuga, S. Ikenoue, M. Tanaka and D. Ochiai. Management of pregnancy after radical trachelectomy. *Gynecologic Oncology*, **162** (2021), 220–5.

10 N. Bhatla, D. Aoki, D. N. Sharma, R. Sankaranarayanan. Cancer of the cervix uteri. *International Journal of Gynaecology and Obstetrics*, **143** (2018), 22–36.

11 A. Ilancheran. Neoadjuvant chemotherapy in cervical cancer in pregnancy. *Best Practice and Research Clinical Obstetrics and Gynaecology*, **33** (2016), 102–7.

12 F. Zagouri, T. N. Sergentanis, D. Chrysikos and R. Bartsch. Platinum derivatives during pregnancy in cervical cancer: A systematic review and meta-analysis. *Obstetrics & Gynecology*, **121** (2013), 337–43.

13. G. S. Leiserowitz, G. Xing, R. Cress, et al. Adnexal masses in pregnancy: How often are they malignant? *Gynecologic Oncology*, **101** (2006), 315–21.

<table>
<tr><td>Chapter</td></tr>
<tr><td>13</td></tr>
</table>

Post-Partum Contraception

Charlotte Gatenby, Catherine Schünmann

13.1 Background

Fertility and sexual activity return quickly following delivery. Just over half of all women in one study (53%) reported resumption of sexual activity and just under half (41%) reported attempting vaginal intercourse within six weeks of giving birth [1–3]. The earliest expected ovulation post-partum in non-breastfeeding women is day 28. Discussions regarding contraception after giving birth have traditionally taken place at the six week check; however, not every woman attends a six week check and contraception may not be discussed or initiated at that visit.

One in 13 women requesting abortion have conceived within a year of a previous birth and 1 in 8 parous women attending maternity services have conceived within a year of a previous delivery [4]. Interpregnancy intervals (IPI), defined as the period from delivery to subsequent conception, of less than 12 months increase the risk of almost all pregnancy related complications, including preterm birth, low birthweight, stillbirth and neonatal death [5, 6]. The World Health Organization (WHO) recommends a 24-month IPI [7].

Sexual and reproductive health strategies across the United Kingdom emphasise the importance of contraception for women after pregnancy [8–10]. Childbirth is a key reproductive event when women are in contact with health-care services and studies show that up to 97% of women giving birth do not wish to become pregnant again in the year following delivery. The immediate post-partum period presents an ideal opportunity to provide contraception for women wishing to avoid an unintended pregnancy and achieve optimum spacing between deliveries [4, 11, 12].

Attending separate providers for contraception when caring for a new baby and recovering from childbirth presents women trying to access timely and effective contraception with unnecessary obstacles that provision immediately after delivery would help to overcome.

13.2 Antenatal Planning for Post-Partum Contraception

13.2.1 When to Have the Discussion

In the context of immediate post-partum contraception, research suggests that discussions relating to contraception and future fertility plans are most usefully conducted antenatally, at approximately 20 weeks gestation. Information in a variety of formats should be made available with a follow-up discussion in the third trimester, in much the same way that mode of delivery is considered and planned following a previous

Caesarean section. If the woman has chosen a method, this should be clearly documented in the handheld maternity record and the best possible effort made by the maternity service to provide this at the time of delivery. If the woman declines all methods, this choice should also be documented and respected. An antenatal plan for contraception provision should be a universal offer and not limited to women deemed to be at greater medical or psychosocial risk from a subsequent pregnancy [13].

13.2.2 How to Have the Discussion

All clinicians providing care for pregnant women should be able to discuss contraception. Pregnant women should be advised of the reliability of different methods including the greater effectiveness of long-acting reversible contraception (LARC) such as subdermal implants and intra-uterine contraception. Clinicians should also ensure that any advice or information given is up to date and accurate and that supporting information can be provided in a variety of languages and formats such as www.contraceptionchoices.org. A holistic approach and shared decision-making should be employed to ensure that women do not feel pressurised into choosing a method they are not comfortable with.

13.2.3 What to Offer

Maternity services should ensure that all women after pregnancy can be provided with the full range of contraception, including the most effective LARC methods, to start immediately after childbirth if desired (Table 13.1). For women who are not fully breastfeeding and who wish to ensure consistent contraceptive cover, a method should be initiated by day 21. Women who cannot be provided with their chosen method of contraception should be informed about services where their chosen method can be accessed. Maternity services should have agreed pathways of care to local specialist contraceptive services (e.g. community sexual and reproductive health (SRH) services) for this purpose.

13.3 Methods of Contraception

The different methods of postpartum contraception are shown in Table 13.1.

13.4 UK Medical Eligibility Criteria (UKMEC)

Clinicians should refer to the UK Medical Eligibility Criteria for Contraceptive Use (UKMEC), which provides recommendations for the safe use of contraceptive methods in women including appropriate methods for women after delivery [14]. It also provides recommendations for women with pre-existing medical conditions or personal characteristics that may present a risk. For each of the risk factors present, which are included in the UKMEC, a category 1,2,3 or 4 is given. It is important to note that the UKMEC does not indicate which method is likely to be most effective, but which methods are safest for that individual. UKMEC categories are not numerically additive in individuals where more than one category applies, but clinical judgement should be used when multiple relative contraindications accumulate.

UKMEC	Definition of category
Category 1	A condition for which there is no restriction for the use of the method
Category 2	A condition where the advantages of using the method generally outweigh the theoretical or proven risks

Table 13.1 Methods of contraception

Method	Main mode of action	Duration	Main benefits	Risks/drawbacks	Failure rate Perfect use (%)	Failure rate Typical use (%)
Levonorgestrel intra-uterine system (LNG-IUS)	Endometrial suppression	3–6 years	User independent Low dose hormone	Invasive, Perforation Expulsion Infection	0.2	0.2
Copper containing intra-uterine device (Cu-IUD)	Gamete toxicity, endometrial hostility	5–10 years	User independent Hormone free	Invasive, Heavy, prolonged bleeds	0.6	0.8
Subdermal implant (SDI)	Anovulation	3 years	User independent	Unpredictable bleeds	0.05	0.05
Injectable Depo-medroxyprogesterone acetate (DMPA)	Anovulation	13 weeks	Moderately user independent	Bone mineral density effect	0.2	6
Combined hormonal contraception (CHC) pill, transdermal patch or vaginal ring	Anovulation	Daily use	Non-invasive Familiar Predictability	Oestrogen – cardiovascular risk – venous thromboembolism, stroke, myocardial infarction	0.3	9
Progestogen only pill (POP)	Anovulation	Daily use	Non-invasive Few risks	Unpredictable bleeds	0.3	9
Male/female condom	Barrier	Immediate	User control Hormone free	Requires planning	2	18
Female barrier, diaphragm or cap	Barrier	Up to 6 hours post intercourse	Female control Hormone free	Requires planning	6	12
Lactational amenorrhoea method (LAM)	Anovulation	Up to 6 months	Hormone free	Requires specific criteria to be met	<2	Not calculated
Fertility awareness methods	Avoidance of fertile phase of menstrual cycle	Immediate	Hormone free	Requires high degree of couple motivation	0.4–5	24

Category 3 A condition where the theoretical or proven risks usually outweigh the advantages of using the method. The provision of the method requires expert clinical judgement and/or referral to a specialist contraceptive provider, since use of the method is not usually recommended unless other more appropriate methods are unavailable or not acceptable

Category 4 A condition which represents an unacceptable health risk if the method is used

13.5 Overview of Contraceptive Method Use in the Post-Partum Period

13.5.1 Intra-Uterine Contraception (IUC)

The levonorgestrel releasing intra-uterine system (LNG-IUS) prevents implantation by maintaining a thin endometrial lining conferring amenorrhoea in up to 70% of women after a year of use. The most widely used LNG-IUSs contain 52 mcgs of levonorgestrel and last five years with a recently released LNG-IUS being licensed for six years. The Mirena® LNG-IUS is also licensed for heavy menstrual bleeding and endometrial protection as part of hormone replacement therapy. Maximal hormonal effect is directed locally within the uterus reducing the likelihood of systemic side effects.

The Cu-IUD is hormone free and acts by promoting an inflammatory response within the endometrium which is hostile to implantation and toxic to gametes. The Cu-IUD can cause heavy, prolonged menstrual bleeding and is chosen less often than the LNG-IUS by women requesting IUC. Both methods are highly effective (failure rate with typical use is 0.2% for LNG-IUS and 0.8% for Cu-IUD) and immediately reversible. The risk of perforation for women who have not recently given birth is quoted as 1–2:1 000. This increases to 6–7:1 000 in post-partum and breastfeeding women if IUC is inserted within six months of delivery. The risk of perforation is also related to the experience of the fitter. Infection occurs with a frequency of 1:20 insertions over the first three weeks of use, thereafter returning to background levels. The risk of expulsion is usually quoted as 1:20 but rises to 1:7 when inserted at Caesarean section or within 48 hours of a vaginal delivery. Routine follow-up at around six weeks post-partum should be arranged for thread checking and this can be managed in an SRH setting. However, although expulsion rates are higher, continuation rates for IUC at six months post-partum are higher in women choosing immediate post-partum insertion than in women undergoing interval insertion, as many in the latter group do not attend for their insertion appointment. Moreover, women choosing immediate post-partum insertion are encouraged to attend for follow-up should they detect signs of expulsion and a high proportion of those women opt for immediate replacement [13,15, 16].

13.5.2 Subdermal Implants (SDI)

The etonorgestrel releasing subdermal implant is inserted over the inner surface of the triceps of the upper arm and gives contraceptive protection for three years. As a user independent method it is highly effective (failure rate 0.05% for both perfect and typical use), immediately reversible and very acceptable to women if inserted immediately post-partum. It acts by suppressing ovulation although it exerts a variable effect on the endometrium and irregular bleeding patterns are a common reason for discontinuation of the method. Approximately 20% of women will experience amenorrhoea with this method, 30% will have regular, light bleeding and 50% of women report irregular bleeding that may be light, heavy or prolonged. Hormonal side effects are commonly reported and SDI use may improve or adversely affect acne. No causal association with mood disturbance or weight gain has been identified from available evidence. It is safe to insert immediately post-partum for any woman (although off licence) and there is no evidence to suggest that bleeding patterns are likely to be influenced negatively by insertion at this time. There is a small risk that implants may be inserted too deeply or migrate along fascial planes. Should the implant become non-palpable, contraceptive efficacy will not be affected but when removal or replacement is due, referral to a specialist service is indicated.

13.5.3 Progesterone Only Injectables – Depo-Medroxyprogesterone Acetate (DMPA)

DMPA is available via intramuscular or subcutaneous routes and is administered either in clinic or by the woman herself at 13-week intervals. It is classified as a LARC (requiring administration less than once per month) but still requires a degree of user dependence which is reflected in the disparity between failure rates with perfect use and typical use (perfect use 0.2%, typical use 6%). Prolonged use is associated with a small reduction in bone mineral density which is reversed on discontinuation of the method. Use of DMPA in women under 18 years who have not reached maximum bone mineral density is UKMEC 2 and therefore, a second-line choice for this reason. DMPA is the only contraceptive method for which there is evidence of weight gain. Women should be advised that weight gain is most likely in those under the age of 18 whose body mass index (BMI) is ≥ 30 kg/m^2. Women who gain more than 5% of their body weight in the first six months of use are likely to continue to gain weight. DMPA can be given immediately post-partum but is categorised as UKMEC 2 in view of the theoretical possibility of a causal relationship between higher dose progestogen and venous thromboembolism (VTE). There is also some evidence to suggest that irregular bleeding may be more common in the immediate post-partum period. However, it is safe and effective for immediate use if first-line methods are contraindicated or unacceptable to the woman. Women should also be advised that although irregular bleeding may be an early side effect, up to 68% of women are likely to experience amenorrhoea after a year of use. Return to fertility on discontinuation of DMPA may be delayed by up to a year.

13.5.4 Combined Hormonal Contraception Including Oral, Vaginal and Transdermal Preparations

Combined hormonal contraception (CHC) acts by inhibiting ovulation, altering receptivity of the cervical mucus and suppressing endometrial growth. In consequence, it can improve dysmenorrhoea and reduce heavy menstrual bleeding. Women should be advised that use of CHC reduces the risk of ovarian and endometrial cancer and may improve acne. Hormonal side effects such as mood change, headaches and weight gain are commonly reported but it is difficult to demonstrate a direct causal relationship based on the available evidence. Oestrogen containing contraception is safe for the majority of women but is associated with a small increase in cardiovascular risk and VTE in particular. The relative risk for VTE is greater with newer progestogens but the overall absolute increased risk remains small. The background risk of VTE for women not using CHC is 2–3 in 10 000 women per year, for women using norethisterone/levonorgestrel/ norgestimate containing CHC it is 5–7 per 10 000 women years and for women using gestodene/desogestrel/drospirenone containing CHC, 6–12 per 10 000 women years. All women should have a risk assessment for VTE post-natally. Women with additional risk factors for VTE should not be prescribed CHC within six weeks of childbirth. These risks include but are not limited to smoking, BMI $\geq$ 30 kg/m^2, Caesarean delivery, post-partum haemorrhage, transfusion and pre-eclampsia.

Women who do not have additional risk factors for VTE and who are not breastfeeding can initiate CHC at 21 days post-partum.

13.5.5 Progestogen Only Pills (POP)

Traditional POPs containing norethisterone and norgestimate act solely by altering cervical mucus. They need to be taken within three hours of the same time every day. The more recently licensed and more widely used desogestrel POP has a 12-hour window and acts by suppressing ovulation in addition to the cervical mucus effect. There are no associations with cardiovascular risk but altered bleeding patterns are common due to the unpredictable effect of progestogens on the endometrium. Approximately 30% of women will have amenorrhoea, 30% may have regular bleeding and the remaining 40% will experience irregular bleeding which may be frequent or prolonged. With continued usage, closer to 60% of women will have amenorrhoea. POPs may worsen acne. Women commonly report symptoms such as weight gain, mood change and headaches although available evidence does not show an association between POPs and these side effects. POPs can be started at any time after childbirth in breastfeeding and non-breastfeeding women.

13.5.6 Lactational Amenorrhoea Method (LAM)

Women who are fully breastfeeding have reduced fertility and breastfeeding is an important method of birth spacing globally. Suckling suppresses ovarian activity but must occur at least four hourly throughout the day and with intervals no greater than six hours overnight to consistently suppress ovulation. Supplementary feeding, use of dummies and expressing may all reduce the effectiveness of this method. Studies have consistently shown that LAM is a highly effective method of contraception with failure rates of < 2% if women are within six months of childbirth, amenorrhoeic and fully breastfeeding. The proportion of mothers who fulfil these criteria in the UK is small and the 2010 Infant Feeding Survey conducted across England, Wales, Scotland and Northern Ireland found that only 17% of women were exclusively breastfeeding at three months post-partum.

13.5.7 Barrier Methods

Male and female condoms can be used at any time after delivery. Female diaphragms and caps should not be used until six weeks post-partum to allow for uterine involution. Women should be advised that the cap size they require may have changed following childbirth. Women at high risk of contracting HIV and women with a previous history of toxic shock syndrome should not use caps or diaphragms. Failure rates with perfect use range between 0.4–5% but are likely to be as much as 1/4 with typical use, due to the high degree of individual motivation needed to ensure correct and consistent use over time.

13.5.8 Fertility Awareness Methods (FAM)

Fertility awareness methods are most effective when multiple indicators are used and have been taught by a trained FAM practitioner. High failure rates are likely with typical use. Insufficient ovarian function immediately after delivery means that this method should not be used until after four weeks post-partum by women who are not breastfeeding, when fertility signs and hormonal changes become detectable again. Woman who are fully breastfeeding are unlikely to have detectable hormonal changes during the first six months post-partum but can use LAM if hormonal or other contraceptive methods are not acceptable and the criteria for LAM are all met.

13.6 Breastfeeding and Contraception

Very small amounts (less than 1% of maternal dose) of contraceptive hormones are excreted in breast milk. A Cochrane review comparing CHC, progestogen only contraception and non-hormonal methods found that the majority of studies did not detect significant differences between methods on breastfeeding duration, breast milk composition or infant growth [17].

Some evidence demonstrates inconsistent effects of CHC on breastfeeding duration, exclusivity and introduction of supplemental feeding and also on infant growth, health and development whether or not CHC was commenced before or after six weeks postpartum. Negative outcomes were not observed with later initiation of CHC. Breastfeeding women who wish to use CHC should be advised that the method can be started from six weeks after childbirth.

IUC and all progestogen only methods can be safely used by breastfeeding women. Studies to date have not demonstrated adverse outcomes on breastfeeding or infant health.

13.7 Initiating Post-Partum Contraception

13.7.1 How Soon Can Contraception be Initiated Post-Partum?

The Faculty of Sexual and Reproductive Healthcare (FSRH) guidance states that: 'A woman's chosen method of contraception can be initiated immediately after childbirth if desired and she is medically eligible' [11]. Although contraception is not required until after day 21 post-partum, it is safe to start all methods immediately except CHC due to increased risk of VTE.

Women who have additional risk factors for VTE in the post-partum period should delay starting CHC until six weeks after childbirth. Similarly, women who are breastfeeding should not start CHC until six weeks post-partum. Women without additional risk factors for VTE and who are not breastfeeding can start CHC from day 21.

IUC can be inserted immediately after delivery and clinicians should be aware that insertion of IUC at the time of vaginal or Caesarean delivery is 'convenient and highly acceptable to women' and is associated with 'high continuation rates and a reduced risk of unintended pregnancy' [11].

IUC can safely be inserted up to 48 hours after childbirth via vaginal or abdominal routes, or at Caesarean section within 10 minutes of delivery of the placenta. There does not appear to be an increased risk of perforation within this time frame. The evidence for safety is limited between 72 hours and 4 weeks post-partum, therefore FSRH guidance recommends that if IUC insertion is not carried out within 48 hours of delivery, it should be delayed until at least four weeks post-partum.

The progestogen only methods (POP, SDI, DMPA) in addition to LNG-IUS can be started immediately after childbirth in women who are either breastfeeding or non-breastfeeding. Although there is no robust causal evidence to link DMPA with VTE, there remains a theoretical possibility that the higher dose and relatively negative effect on lipids of DMPA might be associated with a small increased risk of VTE and so the UKMEC classification is higher for DMPA (UKMEC 2) than POP, SDI and LNG-IUS for use by women within the first six weeks after delivery.

All contraceptive methods are effective immediately if started before 21 days post-partum but extra precautions are required for seven days if a hormonal method is initiated more than 21 days after childbirth. Cu-IUDs are effective immediately, regardless of the timing of insertion.

Table 13.2 shows the UKMEC categories for post-partum women.

13.7.2 Additional UKMEC Conditions

Some women may have medical conditions which pose a significant health risk in addition to post-partum considerations and the UKMEC should be used to aid decision-making in these circumstances. Some conditions of relevance include:

- Hypertension
- Diabetes – type 1 or type 2
- Bariatric surgery within the last two years
- Cardiomyopathy
- Organ failure/transplant
- Sickle cell disease
- Patients using teratogenic medications

13.8 Emergency Contraception in the Post-Partum Period

Emergency contraception (EC) should be considered for any woman who has had unprotected sexual intercourse (UPSI) after day 21 post-partum and who does not wish to conceive. Oral EC can be obtained from pharmacies, primary care and SRH clinics. Insertion of a Cu-IUD for emergency contraception (Em-IUD) can be arranged at SRH clinics and occasionally family doctors. Women contacting pharmacies or primary care who wish to have an Em-IUD should be signposted to their nearest SRH clinic.

Levonorgestrel oral EC is safe to take for women who are breastfeeding. A double dose is recommended for women whose weight is >70 kg or whose BMI >26kg/m^2.

Table 13.2 Summary of UK Medical Eligibility Criteria for Contraceptive Use categories applicable to women after childbirth [14]

Condition	Cu-IUD	LNG-IUS	SDI	DMPA	POP	CHC
Post-partum (breastfeeding)						
0 < 6 weeks			1	2	1	4
≥6 weeks to < 6 months (primarily breastfeeding)			1	1	1	2
≥6 months			1	1	1	1
Post-partum (non-breastfeeding)						
a) 0 < 3 weeks						
With other risk factors for VTE			1	2	1	4
Without other risk factors for VTE			1	2	1	3
b) 3 to < 6 weeks						
With other risk factors for VTE			1	2	1	3
Without other risk factors for VTE			1	1	1	2
c) ≥6 weeks			1	1	1	1
Post-partum (breastfeeding, non-breastfeeding, including post-Caesarean section))						
0 <48 hours	1	1				
48 hours to < 4 weeks	3	3				
≥4 weeks	1	1				
Post-partum sepsis	4	4				

Women who wish to take ulipristal acetate oral EC and who are breastfeeding should be advised to express and discard milk for seven days following administration.

Insertion of an Em-IUD is safe for breastfeeding women from 28 days post-partum and women opting for this method should be counselled regarding the higher risk of perforation for women who are breastfeeding and those within six months of delivery. The Em-IUD will also provide immediate on-going contraception, if this is not desired long term, it can be removed at three weeks after UPSI following a negative pregnancy test.

For further information relating to the correct use of EC, please refer to the FSRH guidance document on EC [15].

13.9 Service Considerations

Immediate post-partum contraception remains elusive in many regions and there are multiple organisational, structural, financial and educational barriers preventing clinicians from providing this service. Routine contraception counselling should feature in every woman's antenatal care pathway and an individualised plan for post-partum contraception should form part of the birth plan. In order to promote informed choice, maternity services should be able to provide IUC and progestogen only methods, including implants, injectables or POP to women before they are discharged from the service. In addition to aligning commissioning to ensure that contraception is easily accessible in secondary care, training and education requirements must also be addressed so that a range of health-care providers feel confident to counsel women about their options and initiate contraception when required. Appropriately trained clinicians including SRH doctors and nurses, obstetricians, midwives, nurses, family doctors and health visitors should be able to provide women with all methods of contraception after childbirth.

Clinical Governance Issues

- An antenatal plan for post-partum contraception provision should be a universal offer and not limited to women deemed at greater medical or psychosocial risk from a subsequent pregnancy
- All clinical staff caring for women in pregnancy should be able to discuss contraception and be familiar with the relevant UKMEC categories
- Maternity services should ensure that the full range of contraception, including the most effective LARC methods, are available to women to start immediately after childbirth if they wish
- Women should be advised regarding the superior efficacy of LARC, but care should be taken to avoid pressuring women into choosing a particular method or indeed any method, if contraception is declined
- Where a woman's chosen method cannot be provided, a bridging method should be offered at discharge until the chosen method can be initiated. Maternity services should have agreed pathways of care to local specialist contraceptive services (e.g. community SRH services) for this purpose
- It is safe to initiate all methods of contraception immediately post-partum except CHC due to increased risk of VTE
- Breastfeeding is not a contraindication to any method of contraception but due to mixed evidence surrounding early initiation versus later initiation, CHC should not be commenced before six weeks post-partum in women who are breastfeeding
- Subdermal implants should be fitted by an appropriately trained provider
- Immediate post-partum IUC should be fitted by appropriately trained providers and a follow-up thread check at around six weeks arranged
- EC should be considered for any woman who has had unprotected sexual intercourse after day 21 post-partum and who does not wish to conceive

References

1 The Scottish Government. *Pregnancy and Parenthood in Young People Strategy.* (2016). www.gov.scot/Publications/2016/03/5858

2 A. R. A. Aiken, C. E. M. Aiken, J. Trussell, et al. Immediate postpartum provision of highly effective reversible contraception. *BJOG: An International Journal of Obstetrics and Gynaecology,* **122** (2015), 1050–1.

3 E. A. McDonald and S. J. Brown. Does method of birth make a difference to when women resume sex after childbirth? *BJOG: An International Journal of Obstetrics and Gynaecology,* **120** (2013) 823–30.

4   R. Heller, S. Cameron, R. Briggs, et al. Postpartum contraception: A missed opportunity to prevent unintended pregnancy and short inter-pregnancy intervals. *Journal of Family Planning and Reproductive Health Care,* **42** (2016), 93–8.

5   C. A. Bigelow and A. S. Bryant. Short interpregnancy intervals: An evidence-based guide for clinicians. *Obstetrical & Gynecology Survey,* **70** (2015), 458–64.

6   G. C. S. Smith, J. P. Pell and R. Dobbie. Interpregnancy interval and risk of preterm birth and neonatal death: Retrospective cohort study. *British Medical Journal,* **327** (2003), 313.

7   World Health Organization (WHO). *Report of a WHO Technical Consultation on Birth Spacing.* (Geneva, Switzerland. 13– 15 June 2007). http://apps.who.int/iris/bitstream/handle/10665/69855/WHO_RHR_07.1_eng.pdf;jsessionid=92FA9B534C99F47B839B91A909CF0A55?sequence=1

8   Department of Health. *A Framework for Sexual Health Improvement in England.* (2013). https://assets.publishing.service.gov.uk/government/uploads/system/uploads/attachment_data/file/142592/9287-2900714-TSO-

9   The Scottish Government. *Sexual Health and Blood Borne Virus Framework 2015–2020 update.* (2015). www.gov.scot/Resource/0048/00484414.pdf

10   Welsh Assembly Government. *Sexual Health and Wellbeing Action Plan for Wales, 2010–2015.* (2010). http://gov.wales/docs/phhs/publications/101110sexualhealthen.pdf

11   Faculty of Sexual and Reproductive healthcare (FSRH). *Contraception After Pregnancy Guideline* (2017). www.fsrh.org/standards-and-guidance/documents/contraception-after-pregnancy-guideline-january-2017/

12   A. Thwaites, L. Logan, A. Nardone, et al. Immediate postnatal contraception: What women know and think. *BMJ Sexual and Reproductive Health,* **45** (2018), 111–17.

13   S. T. Cameron, A. Craig, J. Sim, et al. Feasibility and acceptability of introducing routine antenatal contraceptive counselling and provision of contraception after delivery: The APPLEs pilot evaluation. *BJOG: An International Journal of Obstetrics and Gynaecology,* (2017). https://doi.org/10.1111/1471 – 0528. 14674

14   The Faculty of Sexual & Reproductive Healthcare. *UK Medical Eligibility Criteria for Contraceptive Use (UKMEC).* (2016). www.fsrh.org/standards-and-guidance/documents/ukmec-2016-digital-version/

15   The Faculty of Sexual & Reproductive Healthcare. *FSRH Guideline: Emergency Contraception.* (2017). www.fsrh.org/standards-and-guidance/documents/ceu-clinical-guidance-emergency-contraception-march-2017/

16   R. Heller, A, Johnstone and S. T. Cameron. Routine provision of intrauterine contraception at elective Caesarean section in a national public health service: Aa service evaluation. *Acta Obstetrica et Gynecologica Scandinavica,* **96** (2017),1144–51.

17   L. M. Lopez, T. W. Grey, A. M. Stuebe, et al. Combined hormonal versus nonhormonal versus progestin-only contraception in lactation. *Cochrane Database of Systematic Reviews,* **3** (2015), CD003988.

Further Sources of Information on Individual Contraceptive Methods

www.fsrh.org/standards-and-guidance/documents/ceuguidanceintrauterinecontraception/
www.fsrh.org/standards-and-guidance/documents/cec-ceu-guidance-implants-feb-2014/

www.fsrh.org/standards-and-guidance/documents/cec-ceu-guidance-injectables-dec-2014/

www.fsrh.org/standards-and-guidance/fsrh-guidelines-and-statements/method-specific/combined-hormonal-contraception/

www.fsrh.org/standards-and-guidance/fsrh-guidelines-and-statements/method-specific/progestogen-only-pills/

www.fsrh.org/standards-and-guidance/fsrh-guidelines-and-statements/method-specific/barrier-methods/

www.fsrh.org/standards-and-guidance/fsrh-guidelines-and-statements/method-specific/fertility-awareness-methods/

14

Pregnancy Associated Breast Cancer

Jenna Morgan, Claire Baldry, Emma Ferriman, Lynda Wyld

14.1 Epidemiology of Pregnancy Associated Breast Cancer

Pregnancy associated breast cancer (PABC) is traditionally defined as any breast cancer which occurs during pregnancy or within 12 months of delivery [1] where lactation may be occurring. Some have recently called this definition into question[2], noting that the term PABC should be replaced by breast cancer occurring during pregnancy (PrBC) and a separate category, post-partum breast cancer (PPBC), should be used for breast cancer occurring in the 5–10 years after delivery [2]. Recent evidence suggests that PrBC and PPBC are two distinct entities in terms of biology and behaviour, with PPBC having a worse prognosis [3], although the evidence for this is still in its infancy and more research is needed. For the purpose of this article, the term PABC will be used due to the lack of discrete evidence for separation of PrBC from PPBC in many areas of knowledge. PABC is rare and represents approximately 0.04% of all breast cancers (40 per 100 000 cases) [4] but represents 4% of cancers occurring in women under the age of 45 years and up to 20% of cancers occurring in women between the ages of 25–29 years [5]. Only 1 in 3 000–10 000 pregnancies are linked to breast cancer[5].

The prevalence of PABC is increasing due to the rising incidence of breast cancer generally and the older age at which women chose to have pregnancies in the developed world [6, 7]. A large Swedish study of 1 161 PABC amongst 16 620 breast cancers diagnosed in women under age 44 years found that the rate of PABC increased progressively between 1963 and 2002, from 16 per 100 000 at the start of the period to 37 per 100 000 at the end of the period [5]. PABC generally occurs at a younger age than non-PABC, with the median age being approximately 33 years.

14.1.1 Stage at Diagnosis

Stage at presentation is generally higher in PABC compared to non-PABC. In a large case control study of Japanese women, the time from first symptoms to diagnosis was 6.3 months, one month longer than non-pregnant controls [8]. Stage at presentation was also greater with a PABC stage distribution of 14, 46, 32 and 6.4% for stages 1–4 breast cancer compared to 26, 48, 17 and 1.6% for non-PABC ($p < 0.01$)[8]. The reasons for this are multifactorial and include: lack of screening in this age group; attribution of changes in the breast to the pregnancy by both patients and clinicians; avoidance of mammography to reduce radiation exposure; reduced sensitivity of mammography in very dense, pregnant breast tissue; and the higher prevalence of triple negative and high-grade cancers which may have a pushing border, clinically feeling smooth rather than irregular, implying a benign diagnosis and offering false reassurance.

14.1.2 Disease Biology

The biology of breast cancer is a key predictor of prognosis. Tumour grade and the expression of key tumour receptors (the oestrogen receptor (ER), progesterone receptor and Her-2 receptor) have permitted classification into tumour subtypes with very different prognoses [9]. These include luminal A and B cancers which are both ER positive with good or intermediate prognoses, and Her-2 positive and triple negative cancers, both with poor prognoses.

A systematic review of case series of PABC shows rates of Her-2 positivity to be higher than normal at approximately 33% (in over 955 patients in 18 studies[10]), much higher than rates in the breast cancer population in general, where rates are generally ~15%. In a large Dutch cohort study of 744 PABCs, compared with age matched controls, ER expression was lower in PABC (38.9% versus 68.2%, $p < 0.0001$) and Her-2 receptor expression was higher (20% versus 10%, $p < 0.0001$)[11]. Similarly, triple negative tumours were more common compared to age matched, non-pregnant controls (38 versus 22%, $p < 0.0001$)[11].

Tumour grade is usually higher in PABC compared to the non-pregnant patient, with over 80% of cancers classed as grade 3 in the PABC group compared to 39.5% in a non-pregnant, age matched cohort group ($p < 0.0001$) [11].

14.1.3 Prognosis

Breast cancer associated with pregnancy has a higher mortality and recurrence risk than non-pregnancy associated cancer [12]. The impact of pregnancy may extend well beyond the traditional temporal definition of PABC, with adverse survival outcomes being observed out to five or even 10 years after delivery [2, 13]. A systematic review and meta-analysis of 54 articles relating to PABC reported hazard ratios for overall mortality of 1.45 (95% confidence interval: 1.30–1.63) compared to non-pregnant patients. Disease specific mortality had a hazard ratio of 1.40 (1.17–1.68)[13] in favour of non-pregnant patients. The adverse impact of pregnancy persisted out to 70 months from delivery and indeed may even be worse in PPBC than PrBC [12]. The negative impact of pregnancy on disease aggression is thought to be linked to the biological changes of post-lactational breast involution [2].

14.1.4 Risk Factors

Risk factors for PABC include a greater age at the time of pregnancy; pregnancy over the age of 35 years doubles the risk [7]. There is also a suggestion that Caesarean delivery may increase the risk of breast cancer although the increase in risk was not great and was not statistically significant (HR 1.24, 95% CI 0.98–1.55)[7]. It was not clear whether this was a causal association. Primiparity was found to have a protective effect, although this may have been confounded by age. Whilst it is accepted that pregnancy itself, especially if at a young age, and followed by breastfeeding, protects against the development of breast cancer later in life, there is some evidence that in the early post-partum years, the risk of developing breast cancer is elevated, with a relative risk in months 7–12 of 1.12 (1.01–1.24) and in the second year post-partum of 1.10 (1.03–1.18) [14]. A Norwegian study of over 800 000 women also found that pregnancy was linked to a short-term increase in the risk of breast cancer, which peaked 3–4 years after delivery [15].

In women who carry pathogenic BRCA 1 or 2 mutations, pregnancy does not have a protective effect and may increase the risk of developing breast cancer [16, 17].

14.2 Diagnosis

Due to a lack of routine screening in this age group women with PABC present symptomatically, usually with a breast lump. Due to the age profile of this group of women the most common causes of breast lumps are fibrocystic change, fibroadenomas, galactoceles and infections. Triple assessment should still be performed with clinical examination, ultrasound scanning and core biopsy. Mammography is not typically performed until after confirmation of a cancer diagnosis or if the degree of clinical suspicion is high. Ultrasound has a high sensitivity and is very good at characterisation of benign breast masses, however biopsy is still required in most cases [18]. The X-ray dose of standard mammography is not high and represents the equivalent of seven weeks of background radiation, with a dose to the uterus of only 0.03 microGy, which is well below the 50 microGy threshold associated with a risk of fetal damage [19]. Use of shielding with a lead apron reduces this by 50% [20]. The sensitivity of mammography is lower due to the young age of the patient and the impact of pregnancy associated hormonal changes increasing breast density [19]. In a lactating woman, the breast may be disengorged by the use of a breast pump or breastfeeding just before imaging, which may also make the procedure more comfortable [21]. MRI of the breast, used to diagnose or stage breast cancer, should be avoided during pregnancy as gadolinium crosses the placental barrier and may be harmful to the fetus [20], although it is safe during lactation [21]. Core biopsy is safe, although in a patient who is lactating there is a small risk of creating a milk fistula and therefore, the smallest gauge needle should be used and the breast should be suckled or pumped beforehand to disengorge [20]. For women who are lactating and require biopsies or surgery, rapid suppression of lactation may be achieved with cabergoline before biopsies or surgery are performed, to reduce the risk of lactational fistulae.

If staging is required, a chest X-ray (with abdominal shielding) and liver ultrasound should be advised instead of a CT scan.

It is essential to inform the pathologist that the patient is pregnant when sending biopsies, otherwise the proliferative changes of pregnancy may cause diagnostic confusion.

Lastly, the case should be reviewed at a properly constituted multidisciplinary team (MDT) to confirm the diagnosis and, in cases of pregnancy, this review should include an obstetrician and in some cases a neonatologist.

14.2.1 Pregnancy Termination

Sensitive discussion about the future of the pregnancy should be had in conjunction with the wider MDT taking into account the patients' wishes, prognosis, treatment requirements and impacts on future fertility [22]. Some women may wish to terminate, whilst some may feel the pregnancy is even more precious, in view of the threat to future fertility if chemotherapy is required.

Termination does not improve prognosis but may facilitate therapies. Early engagement with obstetrics to confirm the health and stage of the pregnancy, and regular close obstetric follow-up is essential. Termination may be advised in a woman whose life expectancy is unlikely to see her past the earliest date of viable delivery, as may be the case in a woman with aggressive stage 4 disease (multiple visceral metastases, high tumour burden, cerebral or hepatic metastases and adverse tumour biology). If termination is desired or advised, psychological support for the woman and her partner and family is essential.

14.2.2 Obstetric Management

Ideally, the pregnancy should proceed to full term, but timing may need to be coordinated with other treatments such as chemotherapy. In a large study of pregnancy associated cancer, many of the problems with the infant were actually linked to preterm delivery rather than the cancer therapies [23]. In addition, as most key therapies (surgery and chemotherapy) may be used with relative safety, significant treatment delays should rarely be needed in modern management, with the exception of radiotherapy and anti-oestrogens. The need for radiotherapy may be minimised by use of mastectomy rather than conservation surgery for women where radiotherapy is likely to be delayed by more than three months. Attempts have been made to quantify the impact of treatment delays by use of tumour doubling times and the risk of developing nodal disease and death using mathematical modelling. However, such models make assumptions about tumour doubling times which are not reliably estimated on an individual level, so such models have little clinical value [24]. If early delivery is advised to facilitate treatment, then the mother may be given steroids before surgery to improve fetal lung maturation. Delivery should be managed as normal, ideally a few weeks clear of chemotherapy either way (to reduce the risk of bleeding and infection).

Placental metastases from breast cancer are exceptionally rare, only being seen with highly aggressive tumours, with less than 100 cases reported in global literature and no cases reported where the infant has been affected with the cancer [25].

14.3 Treatment

Management of breast cancer in pregnancy is complex and depends on disease stage, biology and gestational age of the pregnancy and is summarised in Figure 14.1. The mainstays of therapy are surgery to the breast and axilla, adjuvant radiotherapy to the breast or chest wall and a range of systemic therapies including chemotherapy, anti-oestrogens and Her-2 targeting agents (trastuzumab, pertuzumab, neratinib and trastuzumab emtansine). Treatment is tailored to disease biology and stage in normal practice. Schedules are modified to work round the pregnancy and some treatment must be delayed until after delivery. In some cases, to avoid potentially harmful delays in treatment, consideration may be given to early delivery after 34 weeks.

14.3.1 Surgery

Surgery for PABC can safely be performed in all trimesters, although it is important to note that there is a slightly higher risk of spontaneous miscarriage associated with non-obstetric surgery performed under general anaesthesia in pregnancy (reported at 5.8% in one systematic review), with the risk highest in the first trimester (up to 10.5%) [26] and so, surgery is often deferred until the second trimester. This usually does not represent a significant delay when the time taken for the pregnancy to be detected and the time from

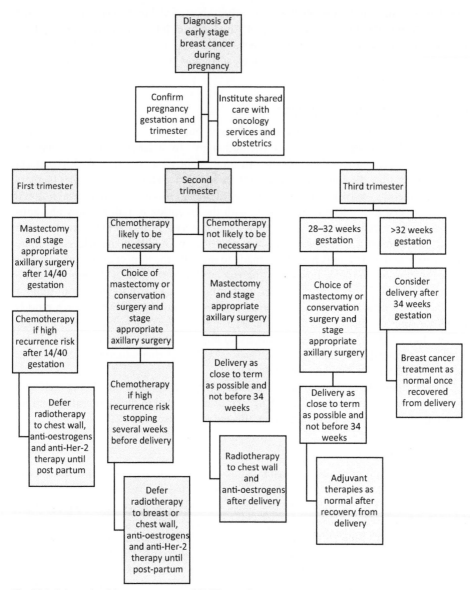

Fig 14.1 Schematic of the management of PABC according to pregnancy gestation

referral to diagnosis are considered. The decision-making surrounding breast conservation versus mastectomy should follow similar guidelines as for non-pregnant patients [27, 28]; however, for those in early pregnancy, the delay to radiotherapy, which cannot be given until after delivery, must be considered. For women who will be offered chemotherapy, this may mean that radiotherapy is not delayed except in women diagnosed in the first or early second trimesters. Evidence suggests that radiotherapy is most effective within three months of surgery [28], and so for those diagnosed in the first and early second trimesters of pregnancy, mastectomy may be considered on this basis, especially if chemotherapy is not planned. For those patients who have mastectomy, immediate breast reconstruction is not recommended as it extends the duration of anaesthesia, with its consequent risk of spontaneous miscarriage. However, there have been a few small series of immediate reconstruction in pregnant patients, showing a short operative time and no significant morbidity to either patient or fetus [29] and so it can be discussed in the context of the limited evidence in this setting – however the surgical technique should be carefully considered, and lengthy autologous flap procedures are best avoided.

For axillary surgery, sentinel lymph node biopsy using technetium-99 radiolabelled isotope for nodal identification can be performed safely during pregnancy [30] but the use of Patent V blue dye to aid node identification is contraindicated due to the risks of anaphylaxis and teratogenicity [27, 31]. Where the use of radiolabelled isotope is not feasible or desired, a four-node sample can be performed as an alternative to sentinel lymph node biopsy in the clinically node negative pregnant patient.

For patients undergoing surgery during pregnancy, it is important that a multidisciplinary approach is used with input from breast surgeons, obstetricians and anaesthetists. Several precautions should be taken including the use of pre-operative steroids for fetal lung maturation in case of inadvertent induction of labour by surgery performed after the time when a viable delivery is possible. The fetus should be monitored continuously throughout the procedure using fetal heart rate monitors. In the third trimester, patients should be positioned with a left lateral tilt to avoid compression on the inferior vena cava by the gravid uterus intra-operatively. Prophylaxis against venous thromboembolism should be undertaken due to the increased risk caused by the pregnancy, cancer and surgery. The breast will be hypervascular during pregnancy and meticulous haemostasis is required intra-operatively to minimise blood loss. If surgery is being performed in the immediate post-partum period, patients should be advised to stop breastfeeding and may require drugs, such as cabergoline, to stop milk production, to reduce vascularity and the incidence of lactational fistulae and sepsis post-operatively. In all cases, obstetric involvement in perioperative care is essential.

14.3.2 Systemic Chemotherapy and Radiotherapy

The principles of non-surgical oncology in pregnancy are the same as for all breast cancers, namely downstaging before surgery (neoadjuvant), treatment after surgery (adjuvant) or to control metastatic disease (palliative). The extra considerations in pregnancy are the risks to the developing embryo/fetus and of complications around delivery.

Cytotoxic chemotherapy is used for most younger women with localised breast cancer. The risk to the mother of inadequate cancer treatment must be considered alongside those of fetal exposure. Risk depends on the stage of pregnancy and the agents used. Pharmacokinetic changes in pregnancy may affect maternal exposure to cytotoxics, although the precise clinical effect of this is unknown [32, 33]. Many cytotoxics are lipid soluble and cross the placenta but transporters such as P-glycoprotein within placental tissue reduce fetal exposure and may account for low levels of observed toxicity *in utero* [34, 35].

Chemotherapy is avoided until the fourteenth week to reduce the risk of fetal malformation and spontaneous abortion [32]. The risk in the first trimester is higher for the combination chemotherapy used in most (neo)-adjuvant regimens, compared to single agents (17 vs 24% in one series)[32, 36].

From the second trimester onwards long-term outcomes are usually favourable and the benefit of treatment usually outweighs the risks, where chemotherapy is a necessary component of the mother's anticancer treatment. Neuropsychiatric and cognitive effects appear to be infrequent and mild, although numbers in most studies are small [37]. Anthracyclines, commonly used in breast cancer, can affect myocardial function, but in a study of 50 children exposed *in utero* there was no evidence of cardiac impairment [37].

Cytotoxic treatment in late pregnancy can cause neonatal myelosuppression. Transient tachypnoea may also occur. Risks to the mother include infection and bleeding around delivery. Chemotherapy is therefore not administered after around 34 weeks of pregnancy [32]. The timing of delivery should be discussed between oncologist and obstetrician.

Patients receiving chemotherapy usually need supportive drugs including anti-emetics, most of which are safe in pregnancy. Granulocyte colony stimulating factor (G-CSF) reduces the risk of febrile neutropenia and observational studies have not shown significant adverse outcomes [38].

Around a third of breast cancers in pregnancy overexpress HER-2 [32]. These cancers are usually treated with antibodies such as trastuzumab. These cause oligohydramnios, possibly by an effect on placental vascular endothelial growth factor (VEGF), or on the fetal renal tubule [39]. The risk of infant death following trastuzumab exposure *in utero* in one meta-analysis was 17% after 25 months follow-up. Exposure early in the first trimester appears to be associated with a lower risk. Therefore, women who become pregnant whilst on these drugs may be able to continue their pregnancy if they stop treatment, but careful counselling is needed [39].

14.3.3 Endocrine Therapy

Endocrine treatment for breast cancer cannot be given in pregnancy. Tamoxifen and its active metabolites have long half lives, so women should not become pregnant for three months after stopping the drug. There is evidence of frequent varied fetal malformations and fetal death with exposure in the first and second trimesters [40]. Hormonal therapy with tamoxifen is associated with oculoauriculovertebral dysplasia (Goldenhar syndrome) and ambiguous genitalia in the neonate [41].

Tamoxifen may increase the risk of clear cell vaginal cancer in female offspring although the evidence is based on animal studies. Aromatase inhibitors may cause labial fusion and ambiguous genitalia in female offspring (Letrozole 2.5 mg film-coated tablets). In premenopausal women, they are always used in conjunction with luteinising hormone-releasing hormone (LHRH) agonists which also cause a theoretical risk of spontaneous abortion and fetal malformation (Zoladex 3.6 mg Implant).

In lactating women, tamoxifen should be avoided, partly because it may inhibit lactation (and indeed was explored as a potential lactational suppressant in the past) [42]. In addition, clinically significant levels of tamoxifen and its active metabolites enter breast milk and may interfere with normal infant development [43]. For most women with ER+ breast cancers diagnosed during pregnancy where anti-oestrogen therapy will inevitably extend into the period of lactation, or in those diagnosed during lactation,

lactation should be stopped (either naturally or with lactational suppressants such as cabergoline) to facilitate anticancer therapies. Many women with PABC will be young and have high-risk cancers and for most therefore ovarian suppressant therapy (gonado-trophin releasing hormone (GnRH) agonists) will be used alongside an anti-oestrogen such as tamoxifen or exemestane. For most with high-risk disease, the duration of anti-oestrogen treatment will be for 10 years. Women wishing to try for another pregnancy during this period will be advised to wait for two years before having a planned holiday from tamoxifen to allow conception and a pregnancy before restarting it.

14.3.4 Radiotherapy

Radiotherapy is always given after breast conserving surgery, and in some patients after mastectomy. Harmful effects include miscarriage, fetal malformation and increased lifelong cancer risk [32, 35]. The doses used are higher than in diagnostic imaging and lead shielding is ineffective. As the uterus enlarges, any dose is likely to be higher, increasing the risk. Radiotherapy is therefore delayed until after delivery.

14.3.5 Future Fertility

A key consideration for some women with PABC diagnosed in the first trimester is whether to continue with the pregnancy. Some women are ambivalent about the pregnancy, perhaps already considering termination before their diagnosis. For others, the thought of dealing with breast cancer and pregnancy at the same time is overwhelm-ing and termination is their choice to allow them to focus on their cancer care. However, when having these very sensitive discussions, consideration must be given to the risk of subsequent infertility due to chemotherapy. The risk of permanent amenorrhoea after chemotherapy varies according to the woman's ovarian reserve (which roughly correlates with age), the type of chemotherapy given and whether ovarian protection is provided by use of agents such as GnRH agonists such as goserelin. The latter may not be used during pregnancy.

14.4 Pregnancy in the Presence of Metastatic Breast Cancer

This is extremely rare. There are three scenarios where this may occur. Approximately 5% of all new breast cancer diagnoses present with metastatic disease, so called *de novo* stage 4 disease. In addition, women with a previous breast cancer diagnosis some years before may get pregnant and then discover that they have metastatic disease whilst pregnant. Lastly, a woman with an established diagnosis of metastatic breast cancer may fall pregnant either accidentally, or, usually against medical advice, as a planned pregnancy. In this latter case, the woman may be on a range of therapies with a significant risk of causing fetal harm. These may include unshielded therapeutic dose radiotherapy, anti-oestrogens, biological therapies, bisphosphonates or chemotherapy. Careful consideration is needed regarding whether the pregnancy should proceed. CT scans are usually performed every 12–18 weeks to assess treatment response for those with metastatic disease, but this cannot be done in pregnancy, so alternative measures of response must be used. Again, timing and mode of delivery need to be managed between oncologist and obstetrician.

14.5 Conclusions

Breast cancer associated with pregnancy and lactation is a challenging problem both for the clinician but also the woman and her family. Close liaison between the breast team (surgeons, medical and radiation oncologists), the obstetric team and neonatal paediatricians, with support from breast care nurses is essential. The aim should be to treat the cancer as fully as possible but with awareness of the limitations imposed by the need to preserve the health of the fetus. In general, the prognosis is less good than for the non-pregnant female, which is largely due to the later stage at diagnosis and adverse disease biology.

Clinical Governance Issues

- Breast lumps are common and usually benign during pregnancy, whereas PABC is rare. However, any woman with a new breast lump during pregnancy must be referred for formal investigation. This should include clinical examination, ultrasound and biopsy
- Mammography with abdominal shielding is safe during pregnancy and may be performed in cases with suspicious breast lumps or where a core biopsy has confirmed cancer. MRI with gadolinium and CT scanning should be avoided during pregnancy
- Management of pregnancy must be overseen by a properly constituted MDT, which must include an obstetrician. A shared care model should be followed
- Consideration of the stage of gestation must be made for all breast cancer treatments, weighing the risk to the fetus against the benefit to maternal prognosis. Whilst many treatments are safe in the second trimester, none are completely risk free and mothers must be counselled accordingly
- Surgery in the second and third trimesters should consider the increased risks of anaesthesia and surgery due to pregnancy with an increased risk of thromboembolic disease, increased risk of bleeding from hypervascular breast tissue, inferior vena cava compression by the gravid uterus and a small excess risk of miscarriage
- Chemotherapy is appropriate in the second and third trimesters with only a small risk to the fetus but should be avoided unless essential in the first trimester and around the time of delivery
- Her-2 targeting agents should be avoided at all stages of pregnancy as there is a high risk of fetal loss
- Tamoxifen should be avoided until after delivery due to the risk of fetal malformation and should be avoided post-partum if the woman is lactating
- Radiotherapy is contraindicated during pregnancy. Doses to the uterus are unacceptably high, even with abdominal shielding
- PABC is emotionally traumatic for the patient and her family and additional specialist support should be provided throughout her care
- The prognosis for PABC is worse than non-PABC and management should reflect this
- Early delivery to facilitate treatment may cause more risk to the fetus than the proposed treatment and should be avoided if possible

References

1   F. Amant, S. Loibl, P. Neven and K. Van Calsteren. Breast cancer in pregnancy. *The Lancet*, **379** (2012), 570–9.

2   F. Amant, H. Lefrere, V. F. Borges, et al. The definition of pregnancy-associated breast cancer is outdated and should no longer be used. *Lancet Oncology*, **22** (2021), 753–4.

3 E. B. Callihan, D. Gao, S. Jindal, et al. Postpartum diagnosis demonstrates a high risk for metastasis and merits an expanded definition of pregnancy-associated breast cancer. *Breast Cancer Research and Treatment,* **138** (2013), 549–59.

4 N. Pavlidis and G. Pentheroudakis. The pregnant mother with breast cancer: Diagnostic and therapeutic management. *Cancer Treatment Reviews,* **31** (2005), 439–47.

5 T. M. Andersson, A. L. V. Johansson, C. C. Hsieh, S. Cnattingius and M. Lambe. Increasing incidence of pregnancy-associated breast cancer in Sweden. *Obstetrics & Gynecology,* **114** (2009), 568–72.

6 L. Knabben and M. D. Mueller. Breast cancer and pregnancy. *Hormone Molecular Biology and Clinical Investigation,* **32** (2017). https://doi.org/10.1515/hmbci-2017-0026. PMID: 28850544.

7 E. J. Kang, J. H. Seo, L. Y. Kim, et al. Pregnancy-associated risk factors of postpartum breast cancer in Korea: A nationwide health insurance database study. *PLoS One,* **11** (2016), e0168469.

8 T. Ishida, T. Yokoe, F. Kasumi, et al. Clinicopathologic characteristics and prognosis of breast cancer patients associated with pregnancy and lactation: Analysis of case-control study in Japan. *Japanese Journal of Cancer Research,* **83** (1992), 1143–9.

9 T. Sorlie, C. M. Perou, R. Tibshirani, et al. Gene expression patterns of breast carcinomas distinguish tumor subclasses with clinical implications. *Proceedings of the National Academy of Sciences of the USA,* **98** (2001), 10869–74.

10 C. F. J. Bakhuis, B. B. M. Suelmann, C. van Dooijeweert, et al. Receptor status of breast cancer diagnosed during pregnancy: A literature review. *Critical Reviews in Oncology/Hematology,* **168** (2021), 103494.

11 B. B. M. Suelmann, C. van Dooijeweert, E. van der Wall, S. Linn and P. J. van Diest. Pregnancy-associated breast cancer: Nationwide Dutch study confirms a discriminatory aggressive histopathologic profile. *Breast Cancer Research and Treatment,* **186** (2021), 699–704.

12 H. A. Azim, Jr., L. Santoro, W. Russell-Edu, et al. Prognosis of pregnancy-associated breast cancer: A meta-analysis of 30 studies. *Cancer Treatment Reviews,* **38** (2012), 834–42.

13 C. Shao, Z. Yu, J. Xiao, et al. Prognosis of pregnancy-associated breast cancer: A meta-analysis. *BMC Cancer,* **20** (2020), 746.

14 T. M. Andersson, A. L. Johansson, I. Fredriksson and M. Lambe. Cancer during pregnancy and the postpartum period: A population-based study. *Cancer,* **121** (2015), 2072–7.

15 G. Albrektsen, I. Heuch and G. Kvale. The short-term and long-term effect of a pregnancy on breast cancer risk: A prospective study of 802,457 parous Norwegian women. *British Journal of Cancer,* **72** (1995), 480–4.

16 H. Jernstrom, C. Lerman, P. Ghadirian, et al. Pregnancy and risk of early breast cancer in carriers of BRCA1 and BRCA2. *Lancet,* **354** (1999), 1846–50.

17 O. Johannsson, N. Loman, A. Borg and H. Olsson. Pregnancy-associated breast cancer in BRCA1 and BRCA2 germline mutation carriers. *Lancet,* **352** (1998), 1359–60.

18 A. P. Ayyappan, S. Kulkarni and P. Crystal. Pregnancy-associated breast cancer: Spectrum of imaging appearances. *British Journal of Radiology,* **83** (2010), 529–34.

19 W. T. Yang, M. J. Dryden, K. Gwyn, G. J. Whitman and R. Theriault. Imaging of breast cancer diagnosed and treated with chemotherapy during pregnancy. *Radiology,* **239** (2006), 52–60.

20 F. Perez, A. Bragg and G. Whitman. Pregnancy associated breast cancer. *Journal of Clinical Imaging Science,* **11** (2021), 49.

21 K. B. Mitchell and H. M. Johnson. Challenges in the management of breast

conditions during lactation. *Obstetrics and Gynecology Clinics of North America*, **49** (2022), 35–55.

22 Royal College of Obstetricians and Gynaecologists. *Pregnancy and Breast Cancer. Green-Top Guideline No. 12.* (2011). Pregnancy and Breast Cancer (Green-top Guideline No. 12) | RCOG

23 S. Loibl, S. N. Han, G. von Minckwitz, et al. Treatment of breast cancer during pregnancy: An observational study. *The Lancet Oncology*, **13** (2012), 887–96.

24 J. Nettleton, J. Long, D. Kuban, et al. Breast cancer during pregnancy: Quantifying the risk of treatment delay. *Obstetrics & Gynecology*, **87** (1996), 414–18.

25 K. Froehlich, H. Stensheim, U. R. Markert and G. Turowski. Breast carcinoma in pregnancy with spheroid-like placental metastases-a case report. *APMIS*, **126** (2018), 448–52.

26 R. Cohen-Kerem, C. Railton, D. Oren, M. Lishner and G. Koren. Pregnancy outcome following non-obstetric surgical intervention. *American Journal of Surgery*, **190** (2005), 467–73.

27 S. Loibl, A. Schmidt, O. Gentilini, et al. Breast cancer diagnosed during pregnancy: Adapting recent advances in breast cancer care for pregnant Patients. *JAMA Oncology*, **1** (2015), 1145–53.

28 A. Toesca, O. Gentilini, F. Peccatori, H. A. Azim, Jr. and F. Amant. Locoregional treatment of breast cancer during pregnancy. *Gynecological Surgery*, **11** (2014), 279–84.

29 V. Lohsiriwat, F. A. Peccatori, S. Martella, et al. Immediate breast reconstruction with expander in pregnant breast cancer patients. *Breast*, **22** (2013), 657–60.

30 O. Gentilini, M. Cremonesi, G. Trifiro, et al. Safety of sentinel node biopsy in pregnant patients with breast cancer. *Annals of Oncology*, **15** (2004), 1348–51.

31 F. A. Peccatori, H. A. Azim, Jr. R. Orecchia, et al. Cancer, pregnancy and fertility: ESMO Clinical Practice Guidelines for diagnosis, treatment and

follow-up. *Annals of Oncology*, **24** (2013), vi160–70.

32 A. E. Ring, I. E. Smith and P. A. Ellis. Breast cancer and pregnancy. *Annals of Oncology*, **16** (2005), 1855–60.

33 G. P. Redmond. Physiological changes during pregnancy and their implications for pharmacological treatment. *Clinical and Investigative Medicine*, **8** (1985), 317–22.

34 K. Van Calsteren, R. Verbesselt, J. Beijnen, et al. Transplacental transfer of anthracyclines, vinblastine, and 4-hydroxy-cyclophosphamide in a baboon model. *Gynecologic Oncology*, **119** (2010), 594–600.

35 F. Poggio, M. Tagliamento, C. Pirrone, et al. Update on the management of breast cancer during pregnancy. *Cancers (Basel)*, **12** (2020), 3616.

36 M. Espie and C. Cuvier. Treating breast cancer during pregnancy. What can be taken safely? *Drug Safety*, **18** (1998), 135–42.

37 S. Esposito, R. Tenconi, V. Preti, E. Groppali and N. Principi. Chemotherapy against cancer during pregnancy: A systematic review on neonatal outcomes. *Medicine (Baltimore)*, **95** (2016), e4899.

38 L. A. Boxer, A. A. Bolyard, M. L. Kelley, et al. Use of granulocyte colony-stimulating factor during pregnancy in women with chronic neutropenia. *Obstetrics & Gynecology*, **125** (2015), 197–203.

39 L. Y. Xia, Q. L. Hu and Q. Zhou. Use of trastuzumab in treating breast cancer during pregnancy: A systematic review and meta-analysis. *BMC Womens Health*, **21** (2021), 169.

40 B. Buonomo, A. Brunello, S. Noli, et al. Tamoxifen exposure during pregnancy: A systematic review and three more cases. *Breast Care (Basel)*, **15** (2020), 148–56.

41 S. L. Cullins, G. Pridjian and C. M. Sutherland. Goldenhar's syndrome associated with tamoxifen given to the mother during gestation. *JAMA: The*

Journal of the American Medical Association, **271** (1994), 1905–6.

42   M. M. Shaaban. Suppression of lactation by an antiestrogen, tamoxifen. *European Journal of Obstetrics & Gynecology and Reproductive Biology,* **4** (1975), 167–9.

43   F. A. Peccatori, G. Codacci-Pisanelli, G. Mellgren, et al. First-in-human pharmacokinetics of tamoxifen and its metabolites in the milk of a lactating mother: A case study. *ESMO Open,* **5** (2020), e000859.

Index